P9-BYT-509

THE OBSESSION

THE OBSESSION

REFLECTIONS ON THE TYRANNY OF SLENDERNESS

Kim Chernin

1817

HARPER & ROW, PUBLISHERS, New York
Cambridge, Philadelphia, San Francisco,
London, Mexico City, São Paulo, Sydney

Grateful acknowledgement is made for permission to reprint the following: "For Ellen West, Mental Patient and Suicide." Copyright © 1981 by Adrienne Rich. Reprinted by permission. Excerpt from "Paying Attention to the Shape We're In." Copyright © 1980 by Carol Shaw. Reprinted by permission. "Tight Denim Jeans" from *Manhattan as a Second Language.* Copyright © 1981 by Jana Harris. Reprinted by permission. Excerpt from *Child of the Dark,* by Carolina Maria de Jesus, translated by David St. Clair. Copyright © 1962 by E. P. Dutton & Co., Inc., and Souvenir Press, Ltd. Reprinted by permission of E. P. Dutton. Excerpt from *Daughter of Earth,* by Agnes Smedley. Reprinted by permission. Excerpt from *Mothers and Daughters,* by Helen Diner. Reprinted by permission of Crown Publishers, Inc. Excerpt from *Winning the Age Game.* by Gloria Heidi. Reprinted by permission of Doubleday & Company Inc. Excerpt from *The Troublesome Helpmate,* by Katharine Rogers. Reprinted by permission. Excerpt from *Adjacent Lives,* by Ellen Schwamm. Reprinted by permission of Alfred A Knopf, Inc. Excerpt from "The Case of Ellen West: An Anthropological-Clinical Study," by Ludwig Binswanger, translated by Werner M. Mendel and Joseph Lyons in *Existence: A New Dimension in Psychiatry and Psychology* edited by Rollo May et al., © 1958 by Basic Books, Inc., Publishers, New York. Reprinted by permission. Excerpted from *Unlearning Not to Speak* by permission of the author. Reprinted by permission of Wallace & Sheil Agency, Inc. Copyright © 1973 by Marge Piercy.

 For information address Harper & Row, Publishers, Inc., 10 East 53rd Street, New York, N.Y. 10022. Published simultaneously in Canada by Fitzhenry & Whiteside Limited, Toronto.

FIRST EDITION

Designed by Robin Malkin

Library of Congress Cataloging in Publication Data
Chernin, Kim.
The obsession.
1. Reducing—Social aspects. 2. Reducing—Psychological aspects. I. Title.
RM222.2.C47 1981 391'.62'0973 81-47224
ISBN 0-06-014884-5 AACR2

---

81 82 83 84 85 10 9 8 7 6 5 4 3 2 1

This book is dedicated to

Susan Griffin

with gratitude for the
inexpressible

CONTENTS

ACKNOWLEDGMENTS

Many people have influenced and encouraged my writing of this book and I am delighted to have an opportunity to acknowledge them.

Susan Griffin suggested that I begin this project and patiently overcame all my resistance to it. She discussed the ideas with me as they were evolving, shared with me her own work on pornography, sharpened my cultural vision, read and edited the final manuscript. The magnitude of the thanks I owe to her must be implied rather than expressed.

Kirsten Grimstadt came across an early version of this manuscript at a time when I had abandoned the project. She encouraged, argued, provoked and finally inspired me back into writing it. She has fought for the book at every stage, in every possible way, has seen it through each successive version and painstakingly sharpened its vision and expression. As an editor and a friend, she has made an invaluable contribution to my life and work.

Roz Parenti read and criticized this manuscript, made important suggestions, encouraged me, believed in me, and shared in every phase of this writing with me. Our friendship, which runs back so many years, has brought me richness and depth and joy.

Michael Rogin read, criticized and encouraged this work as it evolved. Without him it would not be what it has become. Through the conversations, debates and discussions we have shared over many years he has become an essential part of my life and my development.

Lillian Rubin plays a central part in all work I undertake. We discuss everything together and have shared our intellectual and personal lives for many years. I would not be the person I am today without her.

My mother, Rose Chernin, has encouraged me all my life to become a fully developed woman, fully engaged with the world. Her political life, her unflagging energy, and her love for people have been the best possible inheritance to hand on to a daughter.

To my own daughter, my gratitude is due for the understanding she has shown of the many hours I have spent away from her, involved with my work. It is my hope that she will now be able to exercise this same opportunity for self-development fully and capaciously in her own life.

Valerie Miner patiently listened to every word of this book. As a perceptive critic, with a gentle severity and the highest possible standards of style, she has influenced me greatly and has become a dear friend.

Adrienne Rich has given me a careful, detailed, and provocative reading of the manuscript. I have felt deeply the influence of her contribution upon my thinking and writing.

Tillie Olsen argued with me and then guided me toward essential books, the existence of which I would not have known about without her. Her life and work, her presence, and her understanding of "silences" have inspired and sustained me.

At a particularly difficult stage in my writing I came across a brilliant essay by Sandra Gilbert on anorexia nervosa. Her writing proved to be a confirmation of the interpretations I was then formulating. It encouraged and fortified me. Although I did not then know her, I owe her a hearty debt of gratitude.

Luther Nichols was one of the earliest readers of this manuscript. For his support, enthusiasm, and encouragement I cannot say sufficient thanks.

Grace Rutledge performed miracles as a typist. Her quick understanding and perceptive mind made it possible for her to decode all the scribbles and comments written in the margin. For her late nights and early mornings, my deepest gratitude.

My agent, Diane Cleaver, never loses heart. She encourages, believes, advises, and consoles. She was always there when I needed her.

Hugh Van Dusen and Cynthia Merman at Harper & Row are a writer's dream come true. They make the frightening business of a first book's publication seem a joyful and exciting venture between friends. For this I cannot begin to thank them sufficiently.

Finally, my thanks to the women I interviewed and to all those who spoke spontaneously to me about their obsession. For their honesty and courage, their insight and understanding, I shall be indebted for the rest of my life.

The Hunger Song

Hungering, I
go out, I
go ravening into the woods
feed me, I cry
to the trees, desire
rising driven
in me like
a sap and falling
into my body again
I enter into the world
eating the snow, this
is my breath, I
say air of us feeding
me look
at this acorn I made
Love, to know you
like this, flesh
bound as I am, you
in your ecstasy
branching, I
in my green thoughts
growing up
out of the snow.

—Kim Chernin

THE OBSESSION

PROLOGUE

> Food is so fundamental, more so than sexuality, aggression, or learning, that it is astounding to realize the neglect of food and eating in depth psychology. —James Hillman

This is a book about woman's obsession; in particular the suffering we experience in our obsession with weight, the size of our body, and our longing for food. I approach this subject with a sense of personal urgency. I have shared the obsession I am writing about and bring to it only that degree of detachment I have achieved after years of study and thought, my experience interviewing women with a similar problem, and the hours and hours of conversation I have engaged on this topic. Ultimately, the success of this work must depend upon my success as a listener to those almost silent murmurings of my own inner life and to those utterances, frequently whispered, of the women I interviewed and of those to whom I spoke more casually. For our obsession is veiled in shame, profound feelings of guilt, a sense of uneasiness about the behavior of our body and our appetite. When we scratch the surface of this obsession with weight and food we enter the hidden emotional life of woman.

During the nineteenth century woman's experience entered the realm of written and spoken debate. Marriage, domestic labor, child raising, and prostitution, which had not seemed worthy of intellectual consideration, now became serious topics as women began to philosophize about their own condition. In our own time, the female experience of rape, the sexual abuse of female children, the existence of pornography and domestic violence, come increasingly to be examined for the larger meaning in our culture's treatment of women. Thus our sense of what is important and worthy of understanding is enlarged and seriously transformed.

We are, however, only beginning to undertake this examination of deeper meaning where our obsession with food and weight is concerned. Just as we considered rape unmentionable, and abortion shameful, and the subject of domestic labor boring, we have always thought of problems with food consumption as insignificant. Most books written about this subject tell us how to lose or gain weight, how to "firm" the body, how to look beautiful. They do not ask us to become philosophical about the reasons we wish to gain or lose weight. Similarly, psychological thought has slighted the subject of eating and weight (which tend to be women's concerns), just as it has failed to develop a significant understanding of female psychology.

The time has come to break this taboo.

The body holds meaning. A woman obsessed with the size of her body, wishing to make her breasts and thighs and hips and belly smaller and less apparent, may be expressing the fact that she feels uncomfortable being female in this culture.

A woman obsessed with the size of her appetite, wishing to control her hungers and urges, may be expressing the fact that she has been taught to regard her emotional life, her passions and "appetites" as dangerous, requiring control and careful monitoring.

A woman obsessed with the reduction of her flesh may be revealing the fact that she is alienated from a natural source of female power and has not been allowed to develop a reverential feeling for her body.

The body holds meaning. The fact that this thought takes us by surprise itself reflects significantly upon a culture that is seriously divided within itself, splitting itself off from nature, dividing the mind from the body, dividing thought from feeling, dividing one race against another, dividing the supposed nature of woman from the supposed nature of man. As part of this self-division we have come to believe that only those things that concern the soul and the spirit, the mind and its creations, are worthy of serious regard. And yet, when we probe beneath the surface of our obsession with weight, we will find that a woman obsessed with her body is also obsessed with the limitations of her emotional life. Through her concern with her body she is expressing a serious concern about the state of her soul.

This is a book about our veiled and often disguised obsession —with our right to be women in this culture, with our right to grow and develop ourselves and to be accepted by our culture in a way that ceases to do damage to what we are, in our own most fundamental nature, as women.

1. CONFESSIONS OF AN EATER

> What a surprising effect food has on our organisms. Before I ate, I saw the sky, the trees, and the birds all yellow, but after I ate, everything was normal to my eyes. . . . I was able to work better. My body stopped weighing me down. . . . I started to smile as if I was witnessing a beautiful play. And will there ever be a drama more beautiful than that of eating? I felt that I was eating for the first time in my life.
>
> —Carolina Maria de Jesus

> She got up at once, went to get a magnificent apple, cut a piece and gave it to me, saying: "Now Mama is going to feed her little Renée. It is time to drink the good milk from Mama's apples." She put the piece in my mouth, and with my eyes closed, my head against her breast, I ate, or rather drank, my milk. A nameless felicity flowed into my heart. It was as though, suddenly, by magic, all my agony, the tempest which had shaken me a moment ago, had given place to a blissful calm. . . .
>
> —Renée, *Autobiography of a Schizophrenic Girl*

I REMEMBER THE FIRST time I ate compulsively. I was seventeen years old, not yet an introspective person. I had no language or vocabulary for what was happening to me. The issue of compulsive eating had not yet become a matter of public confession. Looking back I can say: "That was the day my neurosis began." But at the time, if I knew the word at all, I would not have known to apply it to myself.

I was in Berlin, sitting at the breakfast table with my American roommate and our German landlords. I remember the day vividly: the wind blows, the curtain lifts on the window, a beam of sunlight crosses the room and stops just at the spout of the teapot. A single, amber drop becomes luminous at the tip of the spout. I feel that I am about to remember something and then, unaccountably, I am moved to tears. But I do not cry. I say nothing, I look furtively around me, hoping this wave of strong feeling has not been observed. And then, I am eating. My hand is reaching out. And the movement, even in the first moments, seems driven and compulsive. I am not hungry. I had pushed away my plate moments before. But my hand is reaching and I know that I am reaching for something that has been lost. I hope for much from the food that is on the table before me but suddenly it seems to me that nothing will ever still this hunger—an immense implacable craving that I do not remember having felt before.

Suddenly, I realize that I am putting too much butter on my breakfast roll. I am convinced that everyone is looking at me. I put down the butter knife. I break off a piece of the roll and put it in my mouth. But it seems to me that I am wolfing it down. That I am devouring it.

I notice, with alarm, that Olga is beginning to clear the table. Unable to control myself, I lurch forward, reach out for another roll and pull the butter plate closer to myself. Everyone laughs and I am mortified. I am blushing the way I have not blushed since I was twelve or thirteen years old. I feel trapped and I want to go on eating. I *must* go on eating. And yet I feel an acute and terrible self-consciousness.

While Olga looks away and Rudi bends over to take something from the mouth of his child, I stuff the two rolls in my pocket, stand up from the table, and leave the room.

Once out of the house I begin running. And as I run I eat. I break the pieces of the roll without taking them from my pocket; I keep the broken portion covered with my hand. Making an apparently casual gesture I raise my hand to my mouth. Smoothly, as if I have practiced this many times, I drop the portion of bread into my mouth. And I continue to run.

Suddenly, as I fly by, I catch a glimpse of myself in the reflecting surface of a store window, looking for all the world as if a tempestuous spirit had been unleashed upon this quiet, bourgeois town. My hair is floating up in wisps, there is something frantic in my face. Perhaps it is a look of astonishment that the body I see there is so very slender when I imagine that it is terribly fat. And then I am violently parted from my own reflection as I race around the corner and stand still for a moment, staring down the street.

I see one of those stations where you can get a sausage, a paper plate, mustard, a white roll. You don't have to enter the restaurant, you can take the thing from an open window, carry it over to a table, stand outside, and dip the sausage in mustard, using your hands. No utensils, no formalities, no civilized behaviors. I slow down and walk up to the window, making every effort to appear at ease. But there is someone in line before me. Suddenly, a wave of tremendous anger and frustration comes over me. I think, if I do not control myself, I shall take this man by the shoulders and shove him aside.

I don't want to wait, I can't wait, I can't bear waiting. I must eat now, at this moment, without delay. I fumble in my pocket for another bit of roll. The pocket is empty. I am kicking at the ground, nudging a small stone about on the pavement. It seems to me, as I become aware of this gesture, that I am pawing the earth. I am terrified now that I will lose control completely—start swearing or muttering or even yelling at the man. I have seen such things before: people who sit speaking to themselves on subways, who burst out yelling for no apparent reason, while everyone laughs. I look down at my coat—it is covered with crumbs. My shoes look shabby. All at once I feel that I am filthy —a gross and alien creature at the edge of unbearable rage. I don't know what to do with myself, the man in front of me still talking to the woman behind the window, his sausage steaming on the counter before him and he does not reach out to take it in his hands. . . .

It is a cold day. I become aware of this as I stand, pawing the ground, watching the steam rise from the sausage. And I know exactly what I am doing when I suddenly dart forward, grab the plate and begin to run. I do not look back over my shoulder, I run with a sudden sense of release, as if I have finally cut the restraint that has been binding me. I hear the man's voice call out. "*Verdammtes Mädel,*" it says. "You damn girl." And then he begins to laugh. I too am laughing as I dart around a corner and stand with my back pressed to a cement building, urgently dipping the sausage into the mustard, stuffing large chunks of it into my mouth. And then I am crying. . . .

And so I ran from bakery to bakery, from street stall to street stall, buying cones of roasted chestnuts, which made me frantic because I had to peel away the skins. I bought a pound of chocolate and ate it as I ran. I never went to the same place twice. I acquired a mesh bag and carried supplies with me, wrapped in torn pieces of newspaper. When I felt tired, I sat down on benches, spread out my food next to me, tried to move slowly, as if I were enjoying a picnic, felt constrained by this pretense, darted the food into my mouth, ran on. . . .

In a few weeks I was planning to return to America. The summer vacation, which had lasted for more than seven months, had finally come to an end. I was out of money; I was tired of traveling, I should have returned home to start college months before. But I knew that I could not go home fat. I looked down at parts of my body—at my wrists, at my ankles, at my calves. There was always something wrong with them, something that could be improved or perfected. How could I know then that the time would never come when I would regard myself as sufficiently slender? How indeed could I possibly imagine that one day I would weigh less than ninety pounds and still be ashamed to go out in a bathing suit? The future was completely dark. I had no idea that this episode of compulsive eating would become a typical event in my life over the next twenty years. It never occurred to me that a whole generation of women would become familiar with this unfortunate experience of their appetites and their bodies, or that I myself would one day weave their experience and my own into a book. At the time my thoughts were riveted upon the shame I felt. I considered going to the movies but I felt so self-conscious that I walked on down the street, feeling that I was a woman of perverse, almost criminal tendencies. I thought that in this obsession with food I was completely alone.

Twenty years later there is laughter. The event has become a story; I tell it to friends and we all smile knowingly. I write it down on the page and I marvel at that young woman running about the streets so frantically, that tempestuous gobbler with her wild eyes. But what has happened during the twenty years? What cycle, beginning that day in Berlin, has now almost accomplished itself, so that today I can sit at my typewriter and dare to look back? Or stand and look at myself in the mirror without considering how I might change this body I see? For it has happened during the last years (and from this I come by degree to believe in miracles) that I have been able to sit down at a meal without computing the calories involved, without warning my appetite about its excess, without fearing what might happen if I took pleasure from my plate. My body, my hunger and the food I give to myself, which have seemed like enemies to me, now have begun to look like friends. And this, it strikes me, is the way it should be; a natural relationship to oneself and the food that nourishes one. Yet, this natural way of being does not come easily to many women in our culture. Certainly it has not come easily to me.

Indeed, if I think back ten years or eight or nine, or to any period of my life, I find that I know exactly how much I weighed, whether I had recently gained or lost weight, exactly what clothes I was able to wear. These facts remain where so many other details have been forgotten. And of course, even in the act of recollection, I hasten to assure anyone who is listening that I was never really fat. Sometimes too slender, I would stand in front of a mirror, practically knocking against my own bones. At other times, when I had gained weight, I would grow attached to a particular pair of blue jeans and Chinese shirt. If an occasion required me to change out of these I felt extremely uncomfortable. These clothes, which I had grown accustomed to, seemed to hide me; anything else I might have changed into would be, I felt, a revelation of how fat I had become. Finally, I acquired a bright colored Mexican poncho; draped in this covering garment, I felt protected from judgments about my immense weight. But that was when I weighed 120 pounds. Surely even the weight charts consider that normal for a woman five feet four-and-a-half inches tall?

During those years my body and my appetite usually inspired me with a sense of profound uneasiness. True, for a week or two after losing weight I would feel that my body had become a celebration. I would rush out and buy new clothes for it, eager to have it testify to this triumph of my will. Inevitably, however, the weight would return. Mysteriously, the willpower would give way to desire. "An extra grape," I'd say, "and I've gained it all back again."

My hunger filled me with despair. It would always return, no matter how often I resolved to control it. Although I fasted for days, or went on a juice diet, or ate only vegetables, always, at the end of this fast, my hunger was back. The shock I would feel made me aware that my secret goal in dieting must have been the intention to kill off my appetite entirely.

When I write about this now it reminds me of the way people in the nineteenth century used to feel about sexuality and particularly about masturbation. I had these same feelings about masturbating when I was a little girl. Then, too, it seemed to me that a powerful force would rise up from my body and overcome my moral scruples and all my resistance. I would give in to it with a sense of voluptuous release, followed by terrible shame. Today, I begin to see that there is a parallel here. A woman obsessed with losing weight is also caught up in a terrible struggle against her sensual nature. She is trying to change and transform her body, she is attempting to govern, control, limit and sometimes even destroy her appetite. But her body and her hunger are, like sexual appetite, the expression of what is natural in herself; it is a futile, heartbreaking and dismal struggle to be so violently pitted against them. Indeed, this struggle against the natural self is one of the essential and hidden dramas of obsession.

Such an understanding did not come to me at all, however, when I was rushing about eating food, or going on diets, or swallowing diuretics, or staring at myself in the mirror, or pinching my waist, or using tape measures to measure the size of my wrists or ankles. For ten or eleven years after that episode in Berlin I felt that my obsession with food and weight was steadily growing more extreme. Finally, I was passing through a period when I found it very difficult to control my eating. Every day, when I woke up, my first thought was about food. Frequently, I could not make it even as far as lunch without eating a pound of candy. When I weighed myself I was filled with alarm by the needle creeping up the scale. "The scale is broken," I would say to myself. "It just wants to pay me back for kicking it," I would explain, not knowing whether or not I actually believed this nonsense. When I went past a mirror I would put my hands over my eyes, frightened of what I might behold there. I even hid from the toaster and the curved surface of a large spoon or the fender of a polished car. In that mood the world seemed filled with reminders that I was not as slender as the woman on the magazine cover, that I, in spite of all my will and effort, was not now able to make myself lean and gaunt.

One night, during this time, I woke around midnight, wondering how I could possibly be hungry, since I had eaten a great deal that day. I lay in bed, hoping I would not get up and go into the kitchen. But I was still hoping this as I made my way down the hallway, walking on tiptoe although I was alone in the house and there was no one to hear me. I opened the refrigerator; there had been a party at my house the day before and much of the food had remained behind. There were, I recall, neatly wrapped packages of feta and grape leaves, a basket of black figs, a few slices of green melon with prosciutto folded across the top, a carefully sliced piece of *boeuf* Wellington, and several chunks of halvah, rising up from a plate of sliced strudel that was flaking off bits of its dough. These were, without question, my most beloved foods and now as I looked at them I was suddenly faced with the necessity of choice. Which should I eat first? I went through several complex computations, persuading myself I would like the halvah better if I ate it after the feta, would not really want the *boeuf* Wellington if I had eaten the strudel first.

In truth, I really wasn't the least bit interested in these foods. Did I want to rush out then and find something in a late-night market? The donut shop perhaps? Or the ice cream store where you could get extra portions of butterscotch? But these foods too seemed to be lacking something. I went to the window of my bedroom and looked out into the garden, trying still to figure out what it was I wanted to eat. But now suddenly, for the first time in my life, I realized that what I was feeling was not hunger at all. I was restless, that was true; I had awakened feeling lonely, I was sad at being alone in the house, and I was frightened: the creaking of stairs, the noise of wind blowing in the window sounded like footsteps to me or like a door opening. What I wanted from food was companionship, comfort, reassurance, a sense of warmth and well-being that was hard for me to find in my own life, even in my own home. And now that these emotions were coming to the surface, they could no longer be easily satisfied with food. I was hungering, it was true; but food apparently was not what I was hungering for.

Recently, I came across a poem which would have helped me greatly if I could have read it years ago. It is by June Jordan and it contains an astonishing insight into the relationship between feeling and hunger:

Nothing fills me up at night
I fall asleep for one or two hours then
up again my gut
alarms
I must arise
and wandering into the refrigerator
think about evaporated milk homemade vanilla ice cream
cherry pie hot from the oven with Something like Vermont
Cheddar Cheese disintegrating luscious
on the top while
mildly
I devour almonds and raisins mixed to mathematical
criteria or celery or my very own sweet and sour snack
composed of brie peanut butter honey and
a minuscule slice of party size salami
on a single whole wheat cracker no salt added . . .

The poem, as it continues, observes the complex social and personal reasons for anger, for loneliness, for the lack of self-love, those emotions which become hunger and rise up from the gut, driving us back to the refrigerator late at night. And it concludes:

Maybe when I wake up in the middle of the night
I should go downstairs
dump the refrigerator contents on the floor
and stand there in the middle of the spilled milk
and the wasted butter spread beneath my dirty feet
writing poems
writing poems . . .[1]

This shift from literal to symbolic understanding is always overwhelming. The poet, distilling the learning of years, dumps out this food that cannot satisfy the complex hunger that is driving her, and stands there writing her poem. And so I learn from her: this hunger I feel, which drives me to eat more than I need, requires more than the most perfectly mixed handful of almonds and raisins. It requires, in whatever form is appropriate, the evolution and expression of self.

Not that this shift to the symbolic will change overnight the way anyone feels about her body or its food. Many times over these years I have continued to wake late at night and have gone back to the refrigerator. I did not dump out its contents. I stood plotting the perfect sequence of food, perplexed at the growing dissatisfaction I felt when I finally began to eat; guilty the next morning, of course, but increasingly driven to reflect upon my experience. For I had the first clue into the resolution of this problem of obsession. I could no longer take it literally. Now, whenever I began to hate my body, or feel fear about the size of my appetite, whenever I began to long for food, I would ask myself what these fears and longings meant.

This research into the meaning of hunger went on for many years, during which I began to talk seriously with other women about their problems with weight. Slowly, it began to occur to me that my understanding of our condition was producing material worthy to become a book. At times, I was excited by this prospect of presenting a careful and detailed analysis of the cultural and psychological meanings of our obsession; at other times I felt that I did not want to continue with this undertaking because its subject matter seemed so trivial to me.

Imagine, I said to myself, spending the next years of your life writing about a woman's problem with her weight. Imagine using all your intellect and all your skill to analyze the reasons for an obsession with food. The obsession had always seemed so petty to me that I could not at times bear the idea that my whole life had already been swallowed up by this preoccupation.

One day, returning from the library, I suddenly realized that this whole idea of triviality was itself revealing. I had been reading Cocteau's book about his addiction to opium and had felt in its writer a distinct sort of pride. "I am speaking of the real smokers," he had written in what seemed to me a remarkably revealing passage. "The amateurs feel nothing, they wait for dreams and risk being seasick; because the effectiveness of opium is the result of a pact. If we fall under its spell, we shall never be able to give it up."[2] I was aware that no woman with a weight problem would make this distinction between the real obsessive and the amateur, for she would see herself, not as a member of an elite fraternity ("the nurses only know the counterfeit smokers, the elegant smokers, those who combine opium, alcohol, drugs . . ."), but as a being afflicted with a dreadful problem she cannot transcend and cannot control. For her, there could be no pride in this, no feeling that her addiction to food exalted her. And yet, Cocteau was able to claim precisely this exaltation for the opium addict. "The addict," he wrote, "can become a masterpiece. A masterpiece which is above discussion. A perfect masterpiece, because it is fugitive, without form and without judges."[3] Opium, I understood, opened the doors to a higher imaginative life; whatever disadvantages the addiction held for the addict, the glamour of this surrender to the higher self placed the addict above the condition of the average mortal. But the woman who surrendered to her obsession with food—who would ever assert this on her behalf? And yet, I reasoned, there must be in this obsession of ours the same deep promptings, the same longings and dissatisfactions, which drove a man to become addicted to opium, to make this pact, to fall under its spell, and never be able to give it up. Our insistence—my own insistence—that our obsession was trivial, was no doubt merely a resistance to what these deeper promptings might reveal.

Some indication of the very great significance of eating can be found in the story of G. T. Fechner, which is told by James Hillman in *The Dream and the Underworld.*[4] Fechner, the founder of psychophysics, was highly regarded by Freud for his work on dreams. But after years of productive work, at the age of thirty-nine, Fechner began to experience a breakdown. His eyes failed and he finally went blind. He also "fell into melancholic isolation, lost control over his thoughts, hallucinated tortures, and his alimentary tract broke down." He remained in this unfortunate condition for three years. Twice, however, he was "miraculously healed: once when a woman friend dreamed of preparing him a meal of Bauerschinken, a heavily spiced raw ham cured in lemon juice and Rhine wine." When she took this dish to him he ate it, against his better judgment, and discovered that his appetite and digestion were both restored. And he was healed also on another occasion when suddenly one morning at dawn "he found that he was able to bear the light and even hungered for it." From this moment his recuperation began, his eyesight returned and he lived on, in good health, for another forty-four years.

As it happened, I was reading this story quite recently in a Berkeley coffee shop. When I looked up from my book I caught sight of several perfectly sliced pieces of Italian rum chocolate cake behind the glass counter next to the espresso machine. I found myself wondering whether I would be able to immerse myself again in the story of old Fechner and prove once more the power of my will to resist my appetite, when the significance of the tale I had just read came home to me. Suddenly, it seemed no accident that Hillman had spoken of Fechner's *hunger* for light. For Fechner, I thought, had been cured precisely by the return of his appetite, when his melancholic withdrawal from the world was superseded by desire. Thus, he begins to eat and his alimentary tract is cured. He begins to hunger for light and his vision is restored. Was it possible, I wondered, that Fechner had been suffering from a severe and controlling attitude towards sensual existence, like so many other intellectual men of the nineteenth century? If so, it made sense that he was healed by giving himself permission to eat, since this permission would have represented a profound reconciliation with instinctual life, a willingness to gratify rather than control desire.

This reflection came upon me as something distinctly new and it made me aware that our obsession had in it as much potential "exaltation" as the surrender to opium. It, too, might be seen as a quest for reconciliation within the self. Opium, perhaps, opened the doors to the higher, imaginative life; but I could now see that our obsession with food expressed a yearning for permission to enjoy the sensual aspects of the self.

This insight had an immediate impact upon my own relationship to food. For the first time in my conscious life I began to imagine appetite as a healthful, natural aspect of myself. I imagined standing up from my table, holding my head high, and walking across the room. In my fantasy I stood calmly in line, not swearing under my breath about the man taking too much time in front of me. Then, I requested the man who worked behind the counter to fill up a tray for me, with two pieces of Italian rum chocolate cake, a large cup of hot chocolate, with espresso and whipped cream. I intended to go sit by myself at a table near the door, letting everyone who passed by look in at me, peacefully eating, not devouring, taking my time, giving myself permission to gratify my appetite.

But now, before I could enact this fantasy, my eyes fell upon the oranges stacked up in an informal pyramid at the top of the counter. The light from the window must have been falling upon them, because they were burnished with a vivid and beautiful glow. I was so fascinated by them that I forgot my conflict about eating; I stared at the oranges, entranced by their roundness. And suddenly I was aware that I had seen them like this when I was a child, on my first trip to California. What a vision that had been as the train passed by the orchard and I shook my mother by the shoulder. "Mama, look," I cried out, waking the old lady drowsing on the seat in front of us, "in California the oranges grow on trees."

This early sense of wonder and delight came to me again now; I looked at the fruit as if it were the gift of a divine being or were itself divine. And now suddenly I realized that my hunger had vanished. I felt that I was being filled with my own joy in the beauty of the world. Everything I looked at now had this same quality of fullness and abundance that gleamed from the oranges stacked in their pyramid across the room. A friend stopped at my table, setting down her tray and bending over to kiss me on the cheek. "You're glowing," she said. "I could practically see you from the other side of the street." She offered me a brioche, which I accepted. But at the first bite I found that I was already satisfied. I took a sip of her coffee, sat back in my chair. "You look," she said, "as if you've swallowed the canary." "Yes," I replied, "I feel as if I'd just eaten the whole world."

For many weeks after that time I found that whenever I was in conflict about food what I needed was permission to eat. If I was in fact able to let myself eat for pleasure, the terrible conflict abated and with it the sense of an insatiable hunger. Frequently, as I observed this conflict over food, I noticed that the permission to eat was closely linked to a delight in life, a sense of joy and abundance, an awareness of some unexpected meaning or beauty. And frequently, too, there were memories of childhood. Occasionally, walking down the street with a salted pretzel from the street stand at the edge of the college campus, I would feel that I had little legs and hands, that I was walking in the Bronx with my mother, tasting everything for the first time. In this state of delight, it never took a great deal of food to satisfy my hunger. However plain or simple it was, to me it seemed exactly the pleasure and satisfaction I had been looking for. The moral to draw from this seemed clear. There was a state of mind and being in which food became a simple, uncomplicated sensual pleasure. But if I were lacking this state, if I simply could not give myself permission to eat, food would not satisfy me, no matter how excellent it was or how much of it I consumed in compulsive rebellion against my own prohibition.

The process of understanding, which over the years was gradually changing my relationship to food, had one last dramatic insight in store for me. This one occurred during a time in my life when I no longer ate compulsively, but would still experience periods of anxiety about my body, feeling that suddenly, overnight I had become fat. On this occasion I was lying in bed counting over the calories I'd eaten during the day. My attention was vaguely focused upon my body, which was filling me with a sense of extreme dissatisfaction. Now, I reverted to a fantasy about my body's transformation from this state of imperfection to a consummate loveliness, the flesh trimmed away, stomach flat, thighs like those of the adolescent runner on the back slopes of the fire trail, a boy of fifteen or sixteen, running along there one evening in a pair of red trunks, stripped to the waist, gleaming with sweat and suntan oil, his muscles stretching and relaxing, as if he'd been sent out there to model for me a vision of everything I was not and could never be. I don't know how many times this fantasy of transformation had occupied me before, but this time it ended with a sudden eruption of awareness, for I had observed the fact that the emotions which prompted it were a bitter contempt for the feminine nature of my own body. The sense of fullness and swelling, of curves and softness, the awareness of plenitude and abundance, which filled me with disgust and alarm, were actually the qualities of a woman's body.

With this knowledge I now got up and went to look at myself in the mirror. For the first time I was able to perceive the transparent film of expectation I placed over my image in the looking glass. I had never seen myself before. Until now, all I had been able to behold was my body's failure to conform to an ideal. Now, I realized that what I had called fat in myself, and considered gross, was this body of a woman. And it was beautiful. The thighs, too large for an adolescent boy, were appropriate to a woman's body. Hips rounding, belly curved, what had driven me to deny this evidence that I was a woman?

For a long moment I stood before my own image, coming to knowledge of myself. Suddenly, I saw all that I was supposed to be but was not—taller, more ethereal, more refined, less hungry, not so powerful, much less emotional, more subdued, not such a big talker; a more generous, loving, considerate, nurturant person; less selfish, less ambitious, and far less given to seeking pleasure for myself.

Now, however, all this came into question: Who, I wondered, had made up this ideal for women? Who had imposed it and why hadn't I seen through it before? Why, for that matter, did I imagine a slender body would bring me these attainments, even if I decided I actually wanted them for myself? And why, finally, wasn't I free simply to throw off this whole coercive system of expectation and be myself—eating, lusting, laughing, talking, taking?

It was a moment of clear vision and it would, I knew, organize the ideas and impressions I had been gathering around a central theme. For now I could no longer doubt that my alienation from my body was the key to understanding my troubled relationship to food, to my appetite, and to my very identity as a woman. I knew also that I would have to go further—to understand, for instance, why so many women of my generation could not tolerate their bodies. I would have to ask why our culture held up before us an ideal image that was appropriate only to an adolescent. I needed to understand whether this inappropriate ideal was part of a much larger coercion exercised against the full and natural development of women.

A book comes into being at that juncture where a personal problem, which has caused great distress, has begun to resolve itself, so that the deeper meanings and wider issues of the problem are apparent. Certainly, I was now beginning to experience a vivid transformation in my way of seeing and hearing. Now, listening to women talk about their problems of weight, I felt myself understanding on many levels at the same time. I went to the same places as before, I listened often to the same women talking, recorded again and again the power of this obsession over their lives, but now I was asking new questions, following different leads, translating everything into a new structure of meaning. And therefore, when a woman said to me one day, "I have rarely had a moment of peace about my body. All my life, no matter what else is going on, I have felt an uneasiness. A sense that something was about to get out of control. That I needed to keep watch. That something about me needed changing," I reached for my notebook and went out to gather evidence that might show how widespread was this uneasiness about the body and its urges. For this obsession, I felt, might well be considered one of the most serious forms of suffering affecting women in America today.

2. THE FLESH AND THE DEVIL

We know that every woman wants to be thin. Our images of womanhood are almost synonymous with thinness.
—Susie Orbach

. . . I must now be able to look at my ideal, this ideal of being thin, of being without a body, and to realize: "it is a fiction."
—Ellen West

When the body is hiding the complex, it then becomes our most immediate access to the problem.
—Marian Woodman

THE LOCKER ROOM of the tennis club. Several exercise benches, two old-fashioned hair dryers, a mechanical bicycle, a treadmill, a reducing machine, a mirror, and a scale.

A tall woman enters, removes her towel; she throws it across a bench, faces herself squarely in the mirror, climbs on the scale, looks down.

A silence.

"I knew it," she mutters, turning to me. "I knew it."

And I think, before I answer, just how much I admire her, for this courage beyond my own, this daring to weigh herself daily in this way. And I sympathize. I know what she must be feeling. Not quite candidly, I say: "Up or down?" I am hoping to suggest that there might be people and cultures where gaining weight might not be considered a disaster. Places where women, stepping on scales, might be horrified to notice that they had reduced themselves. A mythical, almost unimaginable land.

"Two pounds," she says, ignoring my hint. "Two pounds."

And then she turns, grabs the towel and swings out at her image in the mirror, smashing it violently, the towel spattering water over the glass. "Fat pig," she shouts at her image in the glass. "You fat, fat pig. . . ."

Later, I go to talk with this woman. Her name is Rachel and she becomes, as my work progresses, one of the choral voices that shape its vision.

Two girls come into the exercise room. They are perhaps ten or eleven years old, at that elongated stage when the skeletal structure seems to be winning its war against flesh. And these two are particularly skinny. They sit beneath the hair dryers for a moment, kicking their legs on the faded green upholstery; they run a few steps on the eternal treadmill, they wrap the rubber belt of the reducing machine around themselves and jiggle for a moment before it falls off. And then they go to the scale.

The taller one steps up, glances at herself in the mirror, looks down at the scale. She sighs, shaking her head. I see at once that this girl is imitating someone. The sigh, the headshake are theatrical, beyond her years. And so, too, is the little drama enacting itself in front of me. The other girl leans forward, eager to see for herself the troubling message imprinted upon the scale. But the older girl throws her hand over the secret. It is not to be revealed. And now the younger one, accepting this, steps up to confront the ultimate judgment. "Oh God," she says, this growing girl. "Oh God," with only a shade of imitation in her voice: "Would you believe it? I've gained five pounds."

These girls, too, become a part of my work. They enter, they perform their little scene again and again; it extends beyond them and in it I am finally able to behold something that would have remained hidden—for it does not express itself directly, although we feel its pressure almost every day of our lives. Something, unnamed as yet, struggling against our emergence into feminity. This is my first glimpse of it, out there. And the vision ripens.

I return to the sauna. Two women I have seen regularly at the club are sitting on the bench above me. One of them is very beautiful, the sort of woman Renoir would have admired. The other, who is probably in her late sixties, looks, in the twilight of this sweltering room, very much an adolescent. I have noticed her before, with her tan face, her white hair, her fashionable clothes, her slender hips and jaunty walk. But the effect has not been soothing. A woman of advancing age who looks like a boy.

"I've heard about that illness, anorexia nervosa," the plump one is saying, "and I keep looking around for someone who has it. I want to go sit next to her. I think to myself, maybe I'll catch it. . . ."

"Well," the other woman says to her, "I've felt the same way myself. One of my cousins used to throw food under the table when no one was looking. Finally, she got so thin they had to take her to the hospital. . . . I always admired her."

What am I to understand from these stories? The woman in the locker room who swings out at her image in the mirror, the little girls who are afraid of the coming of adolescence to their bodies, the woman who admires the slenderness of the anorexic girl. Is it possible to miss the dislike these women feel for their bodies?

And yet, an instant's reflection tells us that this dislike for the body is not a biological fact of our condition as women—we do not come upon it by nature, we are not born to it, it does not arise for us because of anything predetermined in our sex. We know that once we loved the body, delighting in it the way children will, reaching out to touch our toes and count over our fingers, repeating the game endlessly as we come to knowledge of this body in which we will live out our lives. No part of the body exempt from our curiosity, nothing yet forbidden, we know an equal fascination with the feces we eliminate from ourselves, as with the ear we discover one day and the knees that have become bruised and scraped with falling and that warm, moist place between the legs from which feelings of indescribable bliss arise.

From that state to the condition of the woman in the locker room is a journey from innocence to despair, from the infant's naive pleasure in the body, to the woman's anguished confrontation with herself. In this journey we can read our struggle with natural existence—the loss of the body as a source of pleasure. But the most striking thing about this alienation from the body is the fact that we take it for granted. Few of us ask to be redeemed from this struggle against the flesh by overcoming our antagonism toward the body. We do not rush about looking for someone who can tell us how to enjoy the fact that our appetite is large, or how we might delight in the curves and fullness of our own natural shape. We hope instead to be able to reduce the body, to limit the urges and desires it feels, to remove the body from nature. Indeed, the suffering we experience through our obsession with the body arises precisely from the hopeless and impossible nature of this goal.

Cheryl Prewitt, the 1980 winner of the Miss America contest, is a twenty-two-year-old woman, "slender, bright-eyed, and attractive."[1] If there were a single woman alive in America today who might feel comfortable about the size and shape of her body, surely we would expect her to be Ms. Prewitt? And yet, in order to make her body suitable for the swimsuit event of the beauty contest she has just won, Cheryl Prewitt "put herself through a grueling regimen, jogging long distances down back-country roads, pedaling for hours on her stationary bicycle." The bicycle is still kept in the living room of her parents' house so that she can take part in conversation while she works out. This body she has created, after an arduous struggle against nature, in conformity with her culture's ideal standard for a woman, cannot now be left to its own desires. It must be perpetually shaped, monitored, and watched. If you were to visit her at her home in Ackerman, Mississippi, you might well find her riding her stationary bicycle in her parents' living room, "working off the calories from a large slice of homemade coconut cake she has just had for a snack."

And so we imagine a woman who will never be Miss America, a next-door neighbor, a woman down the street, waking in the morning and setting out for her regular routine of exercise. The eagerness with which she jumps up at six o'clock and races for her jogging shoes and embarks upon the cold and arduous toiling up the hill road that runs past her house. And yes, she feels certain that her zeal to take off another pound, tighten another inch of softening flesh, places her in the school of those ancient wise men who formulated that vision of harmony between mind and body. "A healthy mind in a healthy body," she repeats to herself and imagines that it is love of the body which inspires her this early morning. But now she lets her mind wander and encounter her obsession. First it had been those hips, and she could feel them jogging along there with their own rhythm as she jogged. It was they that had needed reducing. Then, when the hips came down it was the thighs, hidden when she was clothed but revealing themselves every time she went to the sauna, and threatening great suffering now that summer drew near. Later, it was the flesh under the arms—this proved singularly resistant to tautness even after the rest of the body had become gaunt. And finally it was the ankles. But then, was there no end to it? What had begun as a vision of harmony between mind and body, a sense of well-being, physical fitness, and glowing health, had become now demonic, driving her always to further exploits, running farther, denying herself more food, losing more weight, always goaded on by the idea that the body's perfection lay just beyond her present achievement. And then, when she began to observe this driven quality in herself, she also began to notice what she had been thinking about her body. For she would write down in her notebook, without being aware of the violence in what she wrote: "I don't care how long it takes. One day I'm going to get my body to obey me. I'm going to make it lean and tight and hard. I'll succeed in this, even if it kills me."

But what a vicious attitude this is, she realizes one day, toward a body she professes to love. Was it love or hatred of the flesh that inspired her now to awaken even before it was light, and to go out on the coldest morning, running with bare arms and bare legs, busily fantasizing what she would make of her body? Love or hatred?

"You know perfectly well we hate our bodies," says Rachel, who calls herself the pig. She grabs the flesh of her stomach between her hands. "Who could love this?"

There is an appealing honesty in this despair, an articulation of what is virtually a universal attitude among women in our culture today. Few women who diet realize that they are confessing to a dislike for the body when they weigh and measure their flesh, subject it to rigorous fasts or strenuous regimens of exercise. And yet, over and over again, as I spoke to women about their bodies, this antagonism became apparent. One woman disliked her thighs, another her stomach, a third the loose flesh under her arms. Many would grab their skin and squeeze it as we talked, with that grimace of distaste language cannot translate into itself. One woman said to me: "Little by little I began to be aware that the pounds I was trying to 'melt away' were my own flesh. Would you believe it? It never occurred to me before. These 'ugly pounds' which filled me with so much hatred were my body."

The sound of this dawning consciousness can be heard now and again among the voices I have recorded in my notebook, heralding what may be a growing awareness of how bitterly the women of this culture are alienated from their bodies. Thus, another woman said to me: "It's true, I never used to like my body." We had been looking at pictures of women from the nineteenth century; they were large women, with full hips and thighs. "What do you think of them?" I said. "They're like me," she answered, and then began to laugh. "Soft, sensual, and inviting."

The description is accurate; the women in the pictures, and the woman looking at them, share a quality of voluptuousness that is no longer admired by our culture:

> When I look at myself in the mirror I see that there's nothing wrong with me—now! Sometimes I even think I'm beautiful. I don't know why this began to change. It might have been when I started going to the YWCA. It was the first time I saw so many women naked. I realized it was the fuller bodies that were more

beautiful. The thin women, who looked so good in clothes, seemed old and worn out. Their bodies were gaunt. But the bodies of the larger women had a certain natural mystery, very different from the false illusion of clothes. And I thought, I'm like them; I'm a big woman like they are and perhaps my body is beautiful. I had always been trying to make my body have the right shape so that I could fit into clothes. But then I started to look at myself in the mirror. Before that I had always looked at parts of myself. The hips were too flabby, the thighs were too fat. Now I began to see myself as a whole. I stopped hearing my mother's voice, asking me if I was going to go on a diet. I just looked at what was really there instead of what should have been there. What was wrong with it? I asked myself. And little by little I stopped disliking my body.[2]

This is the starting point. It is from this new way of looking at an old problem that liberation will come. The very simple idea that an obsession with weight reflects a dislike and uneasiness for the body can have a profound effect upon a woman's life.

I always thought I was too fat. I never liked my body. I kept trying to lose weight. I just tortured myself. But if I see pictures of myself from a year or two ago I discover now that I looked just fine.

I remember recently going out to buy Häagen Dazs ice cream. I had decided I was going to give myself something I really wanted to eat. I had to walk all the way down to the World Trade Center. But on my way there I began to feel terribly fat. I felt that I was being punished by being fat. I had lost the beautiful self I had made by becoming thinner. I could hear these voices saying to me: "You're fat, you're ugly, who do you think you are, don't you know you'll never be happy?" I had always heard these voices in my mind but now when they would come into consciousness I would tell them to shut up. I saw two men on the street. I was eating the Häagen Dazs ice cream. I thought I heard one of them say "heavy." I thought they were saying: "She's so fat." But I knew that I had to live through these feelings if I was ever to eat what I liked. I just couldn't go on tormenting myself any more about the size of my body.

One day, shortly after this, I walked into my house. I noticed the scales, standing under the sink in the bathroom. Suddenly, I hated them. I was filled with grief for having tortured myself for so many years. They looked like shackles. I didn't want to have anything

> more to do with them. I called my boyfriend and offered him the scales. Then, I went into the kitchen. I looked at my shelves. I saw diet books there. I was filled with rage and hatred of them. I hurled them all into a box and got rid of them. Then I looked into the ice box. There was a bottle of Weight Watchers dressing. I hurled it into the garbage and watched it shatter and drip down the plastic bag. Little by little, I started to feel better about myself. At first I didn't eat less, I just worried less about my eating. I allowed myself to eat whatever I wanted. I began to give away the clothes I couldn't fit into. It turned out that they weren't right for me anyway. I had bought them with the idea of what my body should look like. Now I buy clothes because I like the way they look on me. If something doesn't fit it doesn't fit. I'm not trying to make myself into something I'm not. I weigh more than I once considered my ideal. But I don't seem fat to myself. Now, I can honestly say that I like my body.[3]

Some weeks ago, at a dinner party, a woman who had recently gained weight began to talk about her body.

"I was once very thin," she said, "but I didn't feel comfortable in my body. I fit into all the right clothes. But somehow I just couldn't find myself any longer."

I looked over at her expectantly; she was a voluptuous woman, who had recently given birth to her first child.

"But now," she said as she got to her feet, "now, if I walk or jog or dance, I feel my flesh jiggling along with me." She began to shake her shoulders and move her hips, her eyes wide as she hopped about in front of the coffee table. "You see what I mean?" she shouted over to me. "I love it."

This image of a woman dancing came with me when I sat down to write. I remembered her expression. There was in it something secretive, I thought, something knowing and pleased—the look of a woman who has made peace with her body. Then I recalled the faces of women who had recently lost weight. The haggard look, the lines of strain around the mouth, the neck too lean, the tendons visible, the head too large for the emaciated body. I began to reason:

There must be, I said, for every woman a correct weight, which cannot be discovered with reference to a weight chart or to any statistical norm. For the size of the body is a matter of highly subjective individual preferences and natural endowments. If we should evolve an aesthetic for women that was appropriate to women it would reflect this diversity, would conceive, indeed celebrate and even love, slenderness in a woman intended by nature to be slim, and love the rounded cheeks of another, the plump arms, broad shoulders, narrow hips, full thighs, rounded ass, straight back, narrow shoulders or slender arms, of a woman made that way according to her nature, walking with head high in pride of her body, however it happened to be shaped. And then Miss America, and the woman jogging in the morning, and the woman swinging out at her image in the mirror might say, with Susan Griffin in *Woman and Nature:*

> And we are various, and amazing in our variety, and our differences multiply, so that edge after edge of the endlessness of possibility is exposed . . . none of us beautiful when separate but all exquisite as we stand, each moment heeded in this cycle, no detail unlovely. . . .[4]

3. THE SKEPTIC

> She scrambled around until she found the charts that are the real cheaters—you know the kind, don't you? They let you make an allowance for both your age AND your body size. Such charts encourage a very dangerous attitude, by the way, because as soon as you begin to make concessions to age you ARE old.
>
> —Gloria Heidi

> What's so healthy about those skinny underfed models in the slick fashion magazines? Certainly I don't put poison in my body. But I don't damage my mind by starving myself so that I can't think properly. And what's so healthy about dieting so that your face sags and a lot of lines appear right down on your throat and neck? So many people on a rigid diet just look at their waistlines, forgetting that up above they've aged themselves by ten years a lot of the time. That's physical fitness?
>
> —Carole Shaw

AT THIS POINT I would like to raise certain objections that have been inspired by the skeptic in me. She feels that I have been ignoring some of the most common assumptions we all make about our bodies and these she wishes to see addressed. For example: "You know perfectly well," she says to me, "that you feel better when you lose weight. You buy new clothes. You look at yourself more eagerly in the mirror. When someone invites you to a party you don't stop and ask yourself whether you want to go. You feel sexier. Admit it. You like yourself better."

Can I deny these things? No woman who has managed to lose weight would wish to argue with this. Most people feel better about themselves when they become slender. And yet, upon reflection, it seems to me that there is something precarious about this well-being. After all, 98 percent of people who lose weight gain it back. Indeed, 90 percent of those who have dieted "successfully" gain back more than they ever lost.* Then, of course, we can no longer bear to look at ourselves in the mirror. We have to diet again and lose the same five pounds. This time, however, it is more difficult. Perhaps a few pounds go off but now we feel hungry all the time and frustrated. We eat from the moment we wake in the morning. Once again the pounds return.

It is at this point (I tell my skeptic) that the day-dreaming begins, the futile reminiscing, the telling to anyone who will listen about how once we were exactly the weight we wanted to be and all the clothes in the store fit us and all our problems would be solved if only we could become this weight again. But what kind of solution is it, I ask her, to make one's acceptance of oneself depend upon the losing of weight that cannot remain lost? The reason, I say, that 98 percent of women gain back the weight they have lost is simple—that weight belongs to us by nature. We blame our appetites for the regaining of weight; we feel dislike for ourselves; we have the sense that our body is out of control. But the problem is not in the body. It is, rather, in our attitude toward the body.

Having come upon this distinction I hope, of course, that the skeptic has been set to rest. She, however, does not easily grant a point well argued. Filled with uncertainty about this whole process of re-visioning, she leaps forward, finding new difficulties in the argument. "What about health?" she insists. "You know as well as I that obesity is America's major nutritional problem."

Indeed, I, too, used to believe that excess weight causes a problem for health. All the popular magazines and periodicals are filled with this assumption. At first glance it seems one would

*The figures of 90 to 98 percent have become a common citation when people talk about diet and recidivism. I have attempted to elicit such statistics from various diet organizations, who do not seem willing to release them. Susie Orbach (*Fat Is a Feminist Issue*) seems to have discovered the same reticence in them. She refers readers to Aldebaran, "Fat Liberation—A Luxury," *State of Mind 5* (June–July, 1977), p. 34. Readers may also be interested in the KPFA program, "The Politics of Body Size: Fear of Fat," Pacifica Tape Library, Los Angeles, 1980.

have to be crazy to question this cardinal assumption we all share. But even here, where we expect to find unanimity of opinion, it is possible to consider things in a new light.

Dr. Andres is a professor at Johns Hopkins and Clinical Director of the National Institute on Aging. He reports the results of a fourteen-year study of 1,233 people at Northwestern University, in which it was found that the lowest mortality of all his subjects occurred among those who were 24–38 percent "overweight," as defined by the statistical charts. Andres has also reviewed forty studies conducted by other researchers on the relationship between longevity and weight. These studies covered no less than six million people, and ranged from Italian villagers to Helsinki policemen. Andres says: "The populations were extremely diverse, but what's important is that the results all point in the same direction—the desirable weight if you want to live longer has been underestimated. The current chart on doctors' walls, and our own ideas of desirable weight fixed by a sense of aesthetics, are not desirable if you want to live longer."[1]

There is confirming evidence of Andres' survey in another study by Dr. Ancil Keys, the man who developed the K-ration and who is now Professor Emeritus of Physiology at the University of Minnesota. He has found that "in the absence of hypertension [high blood pressure] overweight is not a risk factor at all."[2]

The *Harvard Medical School Health Letter* has recently added its voice to what may well be a new and emerging medical attitude towards overweight:

> For many, being thin is a cosmetic rather than a health goal—which is fine for people who are naturally svelte. But human beings come in a variety of shapes and sizes. It is unreasonable to expect that everyone will conform to a single, ultra-thin standard. A lot of people (especially women) who are not by any reasonable definition overweight are subjected to discrimination and pressure to change their basic body type. This pressure should be resisted,

difficult as it is to do so. Rather than trying to trim their bodies to fit this year's fashions, many individuals should probably cut their clothing more appropriately to their figures.[3]

What does the skeptic have to say about all this? Temporarily, she may be silent. But I, for one, am not willing to be misled by this. The skeptic will return, that we can rely upon. And consequently, let us arm ourselves against her objections with yet another study. The following reflection upon the relationship between the body and health comes to us from a professor of medical anthropology at the University of California at Berkeley.[4]

Dr. Margaret MacKenzie, who has studied the attitudes of various cultures toward the body, first went to Western Samoa in 1976. There, she and her co-workers found some "very heavy people among the adults." Indeed, the women of Samoa tended to gain weight with each pregnancy, becoming increasingly larger over the course of their lives, until by middle age they were by our standards distinctly fat. Being fat, however, is not a problem in Samoa; these large women are admired, they move with ease in their big bodies and it is precisely at this more advanced age that they are permitted to perform those "humorous, almost lascivious" dances upon which travelers frequently comment. But these large women dance without shame, for in their culture there is no social stigma associated with being fat.

Therefore, it is of great scientific interest that these large women of Samoa do not, in spite of their girth, suffer from heart disease or high blood pressure. Indeed, even when they migrate to America, only three out of a hundred immigrants weighing two hundred or more pounds showed any signs of hypertension. And so Margaret MacKenzie asks: "Is it the mechanical fact of being fat which is causing these symptoms, or could it be the experience of being stigmatized?"

This is a poignant idea. The high blood pressure and heart attacks from which our bodies suffer when we are fat may be the result of the shame we feel about our large bodies and may reflect the social condemnation to which these large bodies open us, rather than the inherent, physical dangers of being fat.

Apparently, our shame so afflicts the body that it endures extreme damage to itself, simply because it has transgressed against a cultural standard which may be highly suspect and problematic in the first place.

Dr. George Mann, a career investigator for the National Heart and Lung Institute, has written a searching and informative article on the relationship between obesity and ill health.[5] "The dilemma of fatness for health scientists," he writes, "comes from the conspicuous association of obesity with a number of chronic diseases that appear in middle and old age. It is not so easy to distinguish causation from association in this relation, but it was inevitable that obesity should be taken by the less critical to be the causal agent and to be itself a consequence of sloth and gluttony."

This reflective, philosophically oriented discussion, in the *New England Journal of Medicine,* raises fundamental questions that are frequently not discussed in professional journals. "It is suggestive," continues Dr. Mann, "that weight reduction has rarely been shown to be a useful treatment for any of the chronic diseases."

Apparently, medical science must begin to look beyond its present preconceptions, as Dr. Margaret MacKenzie also suggests. "In particular," concludes Dr. Mann, "there is little to support the widespread dogma of health-education programs that regard obesity as a cause of high blood pressure and treatment of obesity as a useful way of managing high blood pressure."

We do not, however, need to rely upon scientific studies to discover the fact that our obsession with losing weight has nothing to do with a concern for health. The following tale might have taken place in the life of any one of us. It will, I hope, contribute to the skeptic's enduring silence, for it is much more revealing than pages of medical research.

It began a few weeks ago when a friend fell ill. She was taken with severe abdominal cramps. They grew so painful that she was unable to sleep. Although she is a woman used to struggle, capable of endurance, she cried out in pain from these cramps, which were worse, she said, than the contractions of childbirth. In a brief moment of respite, a friend called her on the phone and said in that jocular voice so familiar in our time: "Well, that's a hell of a way to lose weight." My friend was taken to the hospital. There, when the most severe cramps were over and the hospital staff was able to do routine physical tests, a scale was brought into the room. My friend, who had been unable to eat for several days, felt distinctly happy to see that scale. "I jumped off the bed," she told me, "I ran over to it. 'What's it say, what's it say?' I kept asking the attendants. And then, when they told me, I repeated triumphantly: 'I've lost four and a half pounds.' "

When she was discharged from the hospital, with the condition undiagnosed but possibly abdominal cancer, my friend came home. There, the first thing she did was to rush into the bathroom and go over to the scale.

"I'd like to tell you," she said to me, "that I'd willingly gain back the five pounds rather than go through that horrible pain again. But I honestly don't know whether that's true."

Thanksgiving arrived. After dinner, another very close friend, whose affection cannot be doubted, threw her arms around the woman who had been ill. "Well," she said to her, "at least there's a bright side to this whole thing. You've managed to lose five pounds." Another friend, to whom this saga was told, confessed: "I didn't want to say anything, but I was thinking the same thing myself. After all, you have managed to lose five pounds."

None of these women is an example of psychological derangement. By all the standards used to measure mental adjustment in our culture, they measure up well. They are professional women, able to combine family life and careers, women who have raised or are raising children, women with a capacity for life and joy, close and meaningful friendship. The fact that they all suffer from this obsession, longing for slenderness even at the expense of health, casts no lurid light upon them. It casts rather a highly revealing beam upon our condition as women in our culture today.

But the skeptic who wakes in one's own brain is a formidable opponent; she would prefer that I see this issue the way I have always seen it, ignoring my plea that we re-examine everything we have ever thought about the body. "We all know there are obese people in this country," she now cries out. "Are you trying to argue that fact out of existence?"

Granted, I say, there are obese people in this country. But I am concerned here with the large numbers of us who think we are overweight when we are not and spend the better part of every waking moment pursued by a nagging worry about the pseudo-obesity we suffer from. "Well over half the women I meet," writes Lillian Rubin in her deeply perceptive study of middle-aged women, "speak about being fat, say that's the thing they'd most like to change about themselves. Yet, few are anywhere near fat, most not even discernibly overweight. A heavy toll we pay for our national mania for thinness—millions of women whose distorted perceptions of their own bodies give them little peace and rest."

We have entered an era of cultural life when everyone is preoccupied with a woman's body but few women, whether fat or thin, feel comfortable living inside the body they possess. What else can it mean that in this country alone some three hundred thousand women have had their breasts enlarged, while another fifteen to twenty thousand women undergo a major operation, every year, to have their breasts reduced?[6]

Since it was founded in the early 1960s,* Weight Watchers has had more than eight million people enrolled in it. This means that every week, across the country, twelve thousand individual classes are held, in which thousands of people, most of them women, discuss their problems with weight. It also means that the women who attend these classes all suffer from the unexamined

*Statistics about Weight Watchers and other diet organizations can be found in *Goldberg's Diet Catalog* by Larry Goldberg, New York, 1977.

idea that there is something wrong with the size of their bodies. The number of women afflicted with this attitude toward their bodies has assumed national dimensions.

DIET WORKSHOP: sixty-four workshops in thirty-one states, Canada and Bermuda. Fourteen hundred groups, forty-five thousand people, meeting weekly to control their weight.

OVER-EATERS ANONYMOUS: fourteen hundred groups where people talk about their problems with their bodies.

THE APPETITE CONTROL CENTER, offering another one hundred groups in New York, Pennsylvania, and Connecticut, where methods are taught to reduce the size of the flesh.

WHY WEIGHT, in Brooklyn, offering its services to one hundred and fifty thousand people who wish to make themselves smaller.

LEAN LINE, INC., with two hundred and fifty locations on the East Coast, to which five hundred thousand people have taken themselves to subdue the flesh.

But the revelations that come to us from the bookseller's list are even more impressive.

Reduce with the Low Calorie Diet: Twenty-five printings since 1953
Dr. Atkin's Diet Revolution: Three million copies in print
The Doctor's Quick Weight Loss Diet: Five million copies sold
The Cheater's Diet: Five hundred million purse books sold

There are dozens and dozens of books and organizations, ministering to the needs of millions of people, most of them women. There are countless camps, spas, health resorts, and farms where people pay between $185.00 and $3,000.00 a week[7] in the pursuit of this apparently unattainable and illusory condition of an acceptable body. In this era, when inflation has assumed alarming proportions and the threat of nuclear war has become a serious danger, when violent crime is on the increase and unemployment a persistent social fact, five hundred people are asked by the pollsters what they fear most in the world and one hundred and ninety of them answer that their greatest fear is "getting fat."[8] Indeed, in our land today, twenty million people are on a "serious" diet at any moment.[9] Between them they are spending over ten billion dollars each year in the effort to take weight off and keep it away.[10]

Here, of course, we might expect the skeptic to object, reminding us that 46 percent of Americans are overweight* and that this figure justifies the number of books sold, the billions of dollars spent, the hours invested in this enterprise of changing the size and shape of the body. But the skeptic has passed from silence to curiosity. She is interested in what is being argued here and with a new eagerness is willing to reflect upon the meanings hidden in the statistical chart. For if we accept the reasoning of Dr. Andres (and Dr. Keys, and the *Harvard Medical School Health Letter*) and follow the revised weight charts Andres has proposed, we are all now permitted to gain fifteen pounds or even more in the interest of health. Thus, the medical justification for this preoccupation with the body vanishes. The statistic of 46% can no longer be maintained. Even the insurance companies begin to raise their standards of permissible weight. And we are left to wonder what strange game we are playing when we assure ourselves that America's greatest nutritional problem is obesity.

Science is not neutral in its judgments, nor dispassionate, nor detached; and this fact becomes apparent when we take over the role of skeptic on our own behalf and begin to question the prominent assumptions of our culture.

"What we're dealing with," says Margaret MacKenzie, "is not an unbiased, objective science. The experiments may in fact be carried out immaculately once the hypotheses are phrased. But

*"According to the Metropolitan Life Insurance Co., 12 per cent of men and women between the ages of 20 and 29 are more than 20 per cent overweight. . . . In the 30 to 39 age group, 25 per cent of American women are more than 20 per cent overweight; from 40 to 49, the figure is 40 per cent, and from 50 to 59, exactly 46 per cent are more than 20 per cent too heavy." *Goldberg's Diet Catalog.*

it's the hypotheses and the theories that tend, again and again, to have moral axioms that go unrecognized and are taken for granted."[11]

It is indeed possible that much of the medical information we have been given about obesity reflects hidden assumptions, moral attitudes, or indeed worries and fears that are disguised by the apparently objective tone of the scientific observer. I, for instance, see a clear parallel between the turn-of-the-century medical view of women's sexuality and today's attitude toward women's bodies. Thus, in 1894 an article appeared in the *Journal of the American Medical Association,* expressing views about sexuality common to its time. "Excessive sexual desire at the menopause," it said, in the cool voice of its unimpeachable authority, "is indicative of disease."[12]

Naturally, since sexual desire was considered an illness, the healing profession concerned itself to discover a cure. And it recommended: ". . . hot douches, gradually increased up to ten quarts daily." That the extremeness of this remedy revealed profound hatred for the idea of sexual desire in a woman, the doctor apparently did not notice. He concluded his article with an observation of his patients' character. "Such patients," he said, "have so much lack of confidence in themselves, their physicians, and their friends, that they have not the willpower to keep up a systematic course of treatment." Here we may breathe a sigh of considerable relief, that these "unstable" women managed, in this way, to avoid the doctor's cure for their sexual appetites.

This voice from the nineteenth century was not, however, a solitary one. It spoke what was the prevailing attitude toward a woman's sensual desire. And it had company, as from this medical book published in 1897, recommending treatments for menopause and noting certain disturbing features of the menopausal experience: "For the congestions of the genital organs, which are sometimes particularly distressing in causing sexual excitement . . . relief may often be obtained by the abstraction of fluid from the *os uter,* either with leeches or by means of puncture with a tenaculum or scalpel."[13]

Certain features of this situation have not changed. Today, feeling an extreme lack of confidence in ourselves, apparently because of our weight, we abandon one "systematic course of treatment" for our appetite after another, go from physician to physician, seek cure after cure. And we lend ourselves to methods and procedures as barbarous and self-punishing as those the worthy doctors of an earlier generation recommended for "treatment" of a woman's sexual desire. Thus, we learn that "a new and highly publicized method for weight control is a procedure of wiring the jaws together . . . while their teeth are braced and wired [the women] subsist on a liquid diet. The braces are loosened once a week so that the teeth can be brushed."[14]

Is it possible then that we today worry about eating and weight the way our foremothers and their doctors worried about women's sexuality?

There is a similar atmosphere—of desperation, of frantic struggle against natural appetite—apparent in the procedures employed at the hundreds of weight and diet clinics that have appeared all over the country. One doctor, whose entire medical practice consists of the effort to help women control their weight, describes his method:

"The program includes injectible methods, low carbohydrate diets, balanced diets, protein sparing and other short-term fasts—along with proper and safe medication . . ."[15] (whatever that might be).

Another doctor offers a twenty-one-day program, treating women with a medication called HCG, Human Chorionic Godadotropin—a "protein hormone . . . recovered from human urine and placentas."[16]

At other clinics "the treatment is never less than 28 days" (twenty-five injections plus three days of diet alone), regardless of the amount of weight loss required.[17]

The tone of these descriptions should fill us with uneasiness.

The degree of exploitation possible, when women are feeling so desperate, is bad enough. But perhaps even more disturbing is that subtle atmosphere of scientific experimentation. Wired jaws, injections of protein hormones derived from urine, use of medications, regimens of exercise and fasting. And all this in the name of what is called health?

In a procedure known as gastric stapling, "two parallel rows of 25 staples are applied by a machine to the top of the patient's stomach, creating a small pouch below the esophagus. A couple of staples are then removed to create a small gap through which food can travel from the esophagus to the center of the stomach . . ."[18]

Dr. William Goodson III, who performs four or five of these operations a month, considers the procedure "experimental." And it has, in fact, the potential for serious repercussions. Like any other surgery on obese patients, gastric stapling can cause clots on the lung, pulmonary problems or pneumonia. "There is also the possibility of injury to the spleen or leaks from the stomach during the course of the operation." Although the staples don't usually leak, says Dr. Goodson III, if they did so postoperatively "it could be fatal."

Ruthe Stein, the reporter who wrote this story for the *San Francisco Chronicle,* described the experience of an obese woman on whom this operation had been performed. A year later this woman again underwent an operation to have eight pounds of excess skin removed from her stomach. Nor indeed would this be the last operation she would undergo in her zealous struggle to reduce the size of her body. She and her physician were planning another procedure which would remove excess skin from her legs. But a week after the first skin operation she fell. While trying to protect her stomach she put her fist through it and opened a wound. The hole in her stomach required further surgical intervention.

Apparently, however, a horror tale like this does not prevent women from seeking these and other similar operations. On the day after this story appeared, Ruthe Stein received a large number of calls from women eager to find out where such operations, with all their dangers, could be obtained.

Many of those callers had no doubt been advised by their doctors that their obesity would seriously harm their health. (The obese woman who became the protagonist of Ruthe Stein's story suffered from heart problems. She had once been told that "if she stayed at her former weight . . . she would be in a wheelchair within five years.")

But we know that all doctors do not agree about the effects of obesity upon the heart. And we have seen students of medical research call into question the supposed relationship between obesity and ill health. And we can imagine that this frenzied desire to lose weight is seriously exacerbated by a medical profession which shares with its patients an irrational revulsion for a large body.

In this light it is interesting that the medical profession rarely tells us about the dangers of dieting to excess. The doctors seldom speak about the "chronic fatigue, irritability, tension, inability to concentrate which afflicts chronic dieters."[19] Few cite the findings, also of the medical profession, that it is dangerous to the heart to lose or gain more than ten pounds a year.[20] Few tell us that "without meaningful interruption the chronic anorexic state," to which dieting frequently leads, "may last forever."[21] Few warn about the dangers of electrolyte imbalance, to which the excessive use of laxatives and diuretics may lead. Few talk about just how many women resort to these dangerous methods, in order to comply with the injunctions to be "healthy" and shed that excess weight.

Evidently, the dislike of the body that we have observed in the woman swinging out at her reflection in the mirror influences the medical profession just as it influences the women who flock to the diet organizations, the clinics, and the doctors' offices. It is, apparently, an influential dislike, widespread in our culture.

It can, for instance, be heard clearly in most books about dieting, whether they are written by priests, doctors, nutritionists, fashion consultants, insurance companies, or the establishment. All have a thin veneer of concern for health and for aesthetics, but scratch this surface and you hear a far different order of preoccupation with the flesh.

Just listen: "That swag of flab that swings from armpit to elbow is problem A," the writer says, in her own distinctive poetry of revulsion. "That soufflé of fat that rises between the bra strap and the armpit is problem B."[22] But this utterance seems to have taken on a nightmarish, hallucinatory quality. The hatred for flesh apparently cannot be contained; it spills out, it informs perception, it inflates the horror of what is beheld. The same writer states that it is sad "to see so many stunning women with their beautiful figures spoiled by this great slab of flesh ballooning out over their bra straps." She asks us to share her consternation when viewing one of the legendary Hollywood beauties, with her perfect face and exquisite figure, who turned around and revealed "a veritable Gladstone bag of soft flesh . . . sagging over the top of her low-cut gown and spoiling the illusion."

This is not an idiosyncratic voice. It is, rather, the typical voice of our culture growing lyrical about the horror of fleshly existence. "Being overweight is not just a matter of appearance," says one book; "obesity is a drag, a handicap and a killer."[23] In the event that an individual woman here or there might have managed to escape this obsession, the books warn and admonish. "Fat, obese, overweight, tubby, portly, corpulent, rotund. Call yourself anything you want. You know what you are. It bothers you. It depresses you. And it should frighten you."[24]

It will be profitable for anyone suffering from an obsession with weight to subject these utterances to the same sort of stylistic scrutiny we bring to the analysis of literature, reading them with an ear adjusted to tone and resonance. "You've been warned," says the diet book, "time and time again, what that oppressive extra burden could mean to your health—high blood pressure, heart attack, diabetes . . . early death."[25] Reading this tract I am reminded of the old fire-and-brimstone sermons, intended to frighten men and women away from the delights and pleasures of sexual experience of their bodies. "If you consider," says an early Father of the Christian Church, "what is stored up inside those beautiful eyes and that straight nose, and the mouth and the cheeks, you will affirm the well-shaped body to be nothing else than a white sepulchre; the parts within are full of such uncleanness."[26] In both, the imagery is the same: the white sepulchre of the flesh, the high blood pressure, heart attack, and early death of the overweight.

But there is an immense exaggeration here about the dangers and terrors of overweight, just as in the utterance of the Church Father there was an immense exaggeration about the dangers of a woman's sensual attraction. And this exaggeration allows us to know we are in the presence of some other kind of deeper, less rational worry, having to do with fear and dislike for the body. And so we "learn" that overweight is to be dreaded at all costs. Should one escape serious illness and early death on its account, then, we are told, the very quality of life will be called into question by being fat. "If fat doesn't shorten your life, it surely makes it less rewarding, exciting, worth living."[27] The language of the diet books reveals an urgency of preoccupation that is even more telling than the financial statistics of this industry of weight loss. "You are sentenced to death row in a prison of your own adipose tissue," says one writer, in a style that might have served the great, itinerant preachers of the late Middle Ages in their "diatribes against dissoluteness and luxury,"[28] at which people wept, feared Hell, and did penance for their sins of sensual indulgence.

It does not, I admit, seem at all likely that the women who are attending diet workshops and forming dieting groups and buying this literature of lyrical horror about the dangers of the flesh could possibly be possessed by the same conflicts and worries that caused people in the late fifteenth century to gather by the thousands when a wandering preacher came to town and drove thousands back and forth across Europe, walking barefoot, flagellating themselves, in an effort to atone for venal sins. But the language of these books is certainly suggestive and it cannot hurt us at least to wonder whether our addiction to dieting reveals the same uneasiness about our fleshly existence as inspired those Medieval women and men.

What else, indeed, can it mean that we describe our bodies as a "swag of flab," or a "great slab of flesh," or a "death row of adipose tissue," or a "whited sepulchre containing such uncleanness"?

Surely this language did not issue from people who loved the body.

4. THE HUNGER ARTIST

Whether male or female, patients who don't eat because they don't experience hunger as an appropriate desire have to be taught not only to let themselves eat but also to allow themselves to hunger. —Sandra Gilbert

She must learn again to speak/starting with I/starting with We/starting as the infant does/with her own true hunger/ and pleasure/and rage. —Marge Piercy

FORTUNATELY, the mind is restless; when it uncovers a layer of its own deception, gives up an illusion, exposes a lie, it does not stand idle for long before the collapse of its earlier assumptions. If we wish to know what it is that drives us to make our bodies smaller than they are by nature, we need only turn to some extreme examples of this quest. They will reveal impulses, motives, hidden reasons that operate in all of us but remain hidden, just beyond conscious awareness, precisely because our condition is so much less severe. And it happens that there is a particular group of women who suffer this warfare against the body with unusual severity. These are the girls afflicted with anorexia, a condition in which people starve themselves in order to keep their bodies in a state of skeletal slenderness.

This condition has a peculiar fascination for all of us who diet chronically. And no wonder. For these girls, in their very excess, are living out the logical extension of our shared obsession. Consequently, it is revealing that anorexia is actually an illness that can be fatal.

Dr. Hilde Bruch, who has been studying eating disorders now for more than thirty-five years, tells us that anorexic youngsters "willingly undergo the ordeal of starvation, even to the point of death."[1]

Anorexia is a "self-perpetuating illness," says Dr. Bruch. "It may end in death . . . but more often in painful isolation and chronic invalidism."

Thus, it is of interest that anorexia nervosa, although an illness, has a distinctly exhibitionistic quality—the young people afflicted with it know full well that they can win respect through their ability to display triumph over their bodies. A young woman named Aimee Liu, who has written an autobiographical confession of her struggle with anorexia, leaves us in no doubt about this:

> At lunch my classmates laugh at me for my eccentric eating habits. . . . I lick my spoon at each minuscule bite, and reaching the bottom of the container, insist that I feel full. It is worth it. It wins me notoriety. I'm becoming famous around school for my display of self-discipline. My audience stands in awe of me, and I love it.[2]

Aimee Liu becomes a local celebrity for her demonstrated ability to lose weight. Soon, even the most popular girls at her school come to consult with her as to the secrets of her success. Naturally, she herself admires the type of accomplishment of which she has become such an outstanding avatar. Looking at another girl, whose dress "hangs like a gunnysack on her wasted frame," she speculates about what draws her to her and decides that they share something, "a philosophical standpoint perhaps, a struggle of the will."

This is a crucial insight; and we, who are less extreme in our attitude toward our bodies, can discover from it something meaningful about our own hidden motive to reduce the flesh. Most of us fail, it is true, in every effort to starve ourselves—our appetites return, our bodies grow round again and we resign ourselves to the inevitability of our failure until a new diet appears and the hope is born again that this time appetite can be controlled and the body transcended. But if our will were sufficient to accomplish our desire, many of us would begin to look like our anorexic sister. The anorexic girl has become our present cultural heroine.

It is thus not surprising that Sandra Gilbert calls anorexia nervosa the illness of our decade. "Headlined in the *New York Times* and the *New York Review of Books,* described and discussed in magazines ranging from *Time* and *Signs* to the *Journal of a Woman in Culture and Society,* it is now a glamorous cross between two Victorian favorites, consumption and hysteria, but updated for a modern audience."[3]

This is a revealing description. For these girls, far from being glamorous, are seriously ill; and their illness comes into existence because they, like so many of the rest of us, have taken up an identity with the mind in opposition to the body. As a result, they are pitted against the body and must live out their lives with a determination to inflict their will upon it. Anorexia is, above all, an illness of self-division and can only be understood through this tragic splitting of body from mind.

Hilde Bruch, writing about her anorexic patients in *The Golden Cage,* tells us that "in spite of the weakness associated with such severe weight loss, they will drive themselves to unbelievable feats to demonstrate that they live by the ideal of 'mind over body.' " But most women admire this achievement, we admire the success of their efforts to impose upon the natural body a shape and form which is the product of culture and reflects the power of the mind. Because we are less extreme than the anorexic, this motive toward the body's starvation may escape us when we reflect upon ourselves. But it is the same will to conquer and subdue the body, to adapt it to a cultural standard that is not appropriate for it, that drives our own obsession with the body. We cannot possibly avoid an awareness of this when we listen to the anorexic girls. Unfortunately, this illness is so stereotyped in its expression that when we read about anorexia we seem to be reading the story of a single girl:

"When you are so unhappy you don't know how to accomplish anything, then to have control over your body becomes an extreme accomplishment. You make of your body your very own kingdom where you are the tyrant, the absolute dictator."[4] The girls repeat this idea again and again, in what seems to be the universal monologue of the anorexic condition. Soon, like the rest of us who try to match their efforts, they are driven to test their will by every conceivable means. They refuse to give in to fatigue, they push themselves to swim another lap, perform another difficult calisthenic exercise, run for yet another mile. "Everything becomes a symbol of victory over the body." To be cold with the skin turning blue, although anorexia creates sensitivity to cold, and to deny that one feels cold—this is the typical anorexic posture. "The body and its demands have to be subjugated every day, hour, and minute," we hear. And we are not surprised, then, to read that "many experience themselves and their bodies as separate entities, and it is the mind's task to control the unruly and despised body."

Hilde Bruch tells us how these girls, before the onset of their illness, "were quite definite that they had felt all right about their bodies, pleased for being well-built, tall, and graceful. Some recalled how they had been astonished when other girls expressed concern about their own weight and did something as foolish as depriving themselves. But within a short time, when for whatever reason they began their own dieting ritual, they suddenly looked at themselves differently and could not see they were too thin."[5]

They could not see they were too thin because slenderness had become a statement of power. There could never be too much of it, since more implied that the will had grown even stronger in its relentless struggle to dominate matter.

Behind the glamour of the anorexic heroine we discover thus a desperate and futile struggle. When we look at the anorexic girl, admiring her discipline and asceticism; when we gaze with envy at her as she passes us in the theater, proudly swishing her narrow hips, it is the triumph of her will we are admiring. But we are all so caught up in this struggle against the flesh that we believe we behold beauty in this evidence of the body's emaciation. It is by now, in this culture, virtually impossible for us to see beyond the dictates of this standard. Our obsession has taken possession of our vision of the world. A woman can be neither too wealthy nor too slender, we are told. And we agree. But this vision is an illness we share with the anorexic girl.

Kafka wrote a story about an anorexic, a man so proficient at this conquest over the natural self, in an age so admiring of this achievement, that he became one of the most famous artists of his day.

> Everybody wanted to see him at least once a day; there were people who bought season tickets for the last few days and sat from morning till night in front of his small barred cage; even in the nighttime there were visiting hours, when the whole effect was heightened by torch flares; on fine days the cage was set out in the open air, and then it was the children's special treat to see the hunger artist; [they] stood open-mouthed, holding each other's hands for greater security, marveling at him as he sat there pallid in black tights, with his ribs sticking out so prominently, not even on a seat but among straw on the ground, sometimes giving a courteous nod, answering a question with a constrained smile, or perhaps stretching an arm through the bars so that one might feel how thin it was.[6]

There are times when literature through its heightening and condensation expresses issues that cannot be seen so clearly anywhere else. In this parable Kafka has presented us with a capsule study of the warfare between body and mind that preoccupied his time and seems to have become an even more serious obsession in our own.

The man in the cage is proficient at hunger; he has gathered these large crowds about him through his ability to fast. And here, the extreme pride and sense of accomplishment the anorexic takes in this ability to overcome the craving of natural appetite cannot be in doubt. "For the initiates knew well enough that during the fast the artist would never in any circumstances, not even under forcible compulsion, swallow the smallest morsel of food; the honor of his profession forbade it." Indeed, it is his greatest pain that certain onlookers, nightwatchers who have come to make certain he does not take nourishment, turn aside and provide him with the opportunity to cheat. For this suspicion destroys the whole purpose of his fast, which is intended as a demonstration of his triumph over the body's natural urges. He is glorified by the people who flock to see him because he takes to the furthest extreme the struggle and warfare that is characteristic of his culture.

The hunger artist is celebrated for perfecting a conquest over nature that we all have been educated to accomplish but cannot achieve. The children, of course, observe his deed with special interest, open-mouthed and marveling, because they are still immersed in the learning of this necessary opposition to the body. They, who are still in nature, are praised and loved and cajoled and bullied and intimidated every day of their lives, as they are driven towards this conquest over the natural self. Their wonder testifies to just what a momentous and horrendous accomplishment against nature this is.

Thus, it is a matter of some interest that, in the invented world of Kafka's artist, there is an eventual change in the audience who formerly came to witness this accomplishment. Almost overnight, it seems, a shift in public interest sets in and one fine day the amusement-seekers go streaming past the hunger artist to the cages where wild animals are kept. In the carefully wrought symbolic terms of this story the change in public interest serves to remind us that the admiration for asceticism that we share is not, in fact, a universal condition, but reflects instead particular cultural conflicts. Indeed, the transformation of public sentiment abandons our hunger artist to a famished solitude. It is the wild animals that come now to be admired; people rush past the artist's cage to get to the menagerie. And now, precisely because of this neglect, the artist can fast beyond the limit formerly allowed to him. No one remembers any longer to change the sign that records the number of days of his fast. Soon, he is forgotten.

He lies in grotesque and solitary triumph, bearing witness to a conquest over nature no one admires anymore.

Thus, it happens that when the hunger artist finally starves himself to death, a young panther is introduced into his cage. This panther and the hunger artist stand at opposite poles of symbolic meaning. Where the artist asserts a conquest over nature, warfare against the natural self, and triumph over the body's cravings, the panther is nature triumphant, so powerful in the sheer exercise of being that the caged animal does not even miss its freedom. For this freedom is inalienable, says Kafka, a wild vitality and joy of life in its jaws. And now, everyone feels how "refreshing [it is] to see this wild creature leaping around the cage that had so long been dreary." They brace themselves and do not wish ever to move away.

We, on the other hand, have managed to tear ourselves away. Whatever fascination the panther may once have held for us as a culture, we now hurry past his cage to stand in awe before the new hunger artists of our time. Again, the torches are lighted as the anorexic girl stretches out her slender arm so that we may wonderingly discover how thin it has become. What unites us, performer and spectator alike, in this sorry spectacle of hatred for the flesh, is the shared idea that what the hunger artist achieves is in fact admirable. So far, apparently, it has occurred to none of us that we might set this unhappy warfare aside and love the body instead.

In Kafka's tale, the impresario who travels everywhere with the artist must insist that after a certain time the fast be brought to an end. Experience has proved that the interest of the public cannot be stimulated after forty days. But this loss of interest is something more than boredom. It is evident that after this prolonged period of starvation the hidden meaning of the artist's struggle will become clear. The very extremity of his condition now reveals the inevitable outcome of the warfare against the flesh. It is a battle unto death, with death the only possible outcome. How else can the body be conquered? All the rest of life's purposes must be subordinated to this single, dreadful mania for dominion. Now only the total collapse of the body can testify to the superior power of the will.

But this is horrible, we say; we do not want to see this logical outcome of the struggle against the body in which we, too, are engaged. Better even to have a bit more flesh about us than follow to this fearful consequence our own craving to subdue the body. It is strange, then, that in spite of this insight, we wake the next morning with a peculiar uneasiness about the fact that our body might have grown larger than it was before dinner on the previous night. Strange that we feel this mingled guilt and regret about our appetite, a sense even of shame and despair, as our hand reaches down to feel the hipbone, to measure the curve of the thigh.

And so it happens that we, too, have something to reveal to the anorexic girl. Caged in a cultural ideal of a woman's body, if she should look out at us and wonder what exists beyond the fascination in our eyes, she might suddenly perceive all those negative attitudes toward the body which have closed down the door upon her cage. If it is her destiny to avoid the shame she feels about her body by constantly triumphing over its demands, we, in turn, directly experience that shame. In us she may behold the essential paradox of her own condition, for her pride in the body's conquest is built upon a feeling of profound humiliation that the body exists at all.

When the diet fails, when the dream of conquering our bodies is broken, when the appetite returns and cannot be controlled any longer, the body also returns. The vision of its transformation is shattered and we are aware of this stubborn flesh, in constant rebellion against our will. Then, this body which refuses to jog or lift weights or bend over and touch its toes or swim another lap or eat another mouthful of low-fat cottage cheese fills us with a sense of the most intense despair.

A woman speaks these words. "I can no longer bear to look at myself," she says. "Whenever I have to stand in front of a mirror to comb my hair I tie a large towel around my neck. Even at night I slip my nightgown on before I take off my blouse and pants. But all this has only made it worse and worse. It's been so long since I've really looked at my body. And now it's become, in my imagination, an unbearable grotesque."[7]

What we have heard here is not an isolated voice or an unusual severity. Many of us have known it ourselves and we realize that most women have known it at some time, and there are even further extremes, conditions of despair with the body, when the shame is so great that the body is quite simply and dramatically lost. "Fat people," writes Marcia Millman, "often think of themselves solely in terms of the 'neck up.' Their bodies are disowned, alienated, foreign, perhaps stubbornly present but not truly a part of the real self."[8] And a fat woman says: "I have receded from the physical world."

But this is true for all the rest of us who struggle daily to reduce the flesh; the fat woman and the woman suffering from pseudo-obesity and the anorexic girl have all receded from the physical world. And it follows then that we must begin to experience our bodies as if they were constantly threatening to rage out of control. This is the inevitable result of our struggle to assert the preeminence of our will—this flesh we seek to conquer and subdue now confronts us as an alien from the other side of a division we have created in ourselves.

Because it is nature, the body of a woman grows fuller before the menstrual cycle, takes on water and rounds itself out as if passing through a pregnancy, the blood coming then as if the birth had been aborted, bringing a strangely mixed feeling of release and sorrow. These are feelings that create their own hunger, and so we eat more food before a period, to sustain our bodies as they pass through their crisis and to soothe ourselves in our emotional distress.

Because it is nature, the body of a woman after childbirth grows fuller, the hips grow larger, and the breasts become heavier; with every child the thighs are less like the thighs of an adolescent; a softness comes to our flesh, we grow larger with the body's knowledge of life and of birth. And then later, in menopause, when we begin to round out our lives, we grow more ample than we were before, we are deepened by life and broadened by experience.

These things are according to nature. But we, who have determined to conquer the nature in our bodies, experience these events with alarm. We loathe the swelling in our breasts, the increase in our thighs, we are terrified by the fullness in our flesh. We wear large towels or loose, concealing dresses; we do not go swimming or go anywhere near a dressing room where other women could see the fullness of our breasts and bellies. We hide from ourselves; we deny the seasons of our bodies. They become foreign to us, strangers.

Thus, a woman writes to me about her experience one autumn when she discovers that "the few slacks and shirts she bought last year to accommodate her increasing girth are tight, uncomfortable." She goes shopping and because she knows that she cannot fit into the new fashions she makes her way to the shop that "accommodates the full-figured woman." But now, as she looks in the mirror, she sees that "everything she tries on underscores her metamorphosis. Her reflection in the full-length three-way mirror is more than an embarrassment. It shocks! Who is this stranger? How did it happen? How, why did she allow it to happen, make it happen? She is suddenly panic stricken . . . desperate . . . unutterably depressed. SHE HAS BEEN TAKEN OVER BY HER BODY."[9]

This woman writes of herself in the third person. With this device she distances herself from her own experience of shame and panic, just as in the experience itself, she alienates herself from her body and becomes, as she stares at herself in the mirror, foreign to herself, a stranger. And she, who has such a great appetite for life, leaves my office one day, having talked with much passion and despair about her hatred for her body; and when she hugs me goodbye she turns aside. "I didn't want to press my stomach against you," she says. And then, nervously, unconsciously, as she has done so many times during the last hour, she plucks at the loose blouse she is wearing, pulling it down over this belly she feared would give so much offense.

It is tragic. It is so for all of us. None of us can identify with the hated flesh we are so determined to alter and shape. The most earth-bound of us end by losing the body. Existing from the neck up, we live out our lives feeling alien within it, disembodied.

5. THE OLDEST CULTURAL ISSUE

> The Renaissance insistence upon women's violent and uncontrollable passions, "the unsounded sea of women's bloods," seems related to the belief that woman is less spiritual than man. She is supposed to be less capable than he of controlling lust, gluttony, anger, and greed, because these impulses are stronger in her and reason weaker.
>
> —Katharine M. Rogers

> She didn't fear death itself, welcoming release from her long struggle between mind and body.
>
> —Mary Jane Moffatt and Charlotte Painter

THE BODY troubles us. We find that we cannot be at peace in this body that wakes hungering in the morning, filled with urges and appetites we cannot control and are unable to transcend. But it may help us, in our lonely anguish over the body, to realize that the struggle to dominate the body is endemic to this culture, and may well characterize patriarchal culture altogether. The woman who wakes early, and counts over the number of calories she ate the night before, wondering whether her body has added substance to itself at the expense of her will, is standing within an old tradition.

Norman O. Brown writes:

> For two thousand years or more man has been subjected to a systematic effort to transform him into an ascetic animal. He remains a pleasure-seeking animal. Parental discipline, religious denunciation of bodily pleasure, and philosophic exaltation of the life of reason have all left man overtly docile, but secretly in his unconscious unconvinced. . . .[1]

This old problem, which runs back at least two thousand years in our culture, has assumed in our time an appearance of triviality because of the way it is expressed through a concern with pounds and inches. In other forms, however, it occupied the serious thinkers of earlier times and it continues in fact to exercise the philosophers and psychologists of our own day. Thus, Julian Jaynes attempts to account for the mind/body division by making its arrival in our culture simultaneous with the development of self-reflective consciousness.

> It is now the conscious subjective mind-space and its self that is opposed to the material body. Cults spring up about this new wonder-provoking division between psyche and soma. . . . So Dualism, that central difficulty in this problem of consciousness, begins its huge haunted career through history, to be firmly set in the firmament of thought by Plato, moving through Gnosticism into the great religions, up through the arrogant assurances of Descartes to become one of the great spurious quandaries of modern psychology.[2]

Whether or not we are fascinated by Jaynes' particular idea as to the origins of the body/mind duality, a moment of serious reflection should now convince us that this acute suffering, which daily affects our lives in the form of an unceasing worry about our weight, deserves to be understood in terms of its highly dignified, philosophical antecedents.

Thus, when we learn that all the major Christian writers during the first six centuries of the Christian era "dwelt upon the vexation of marriage and reviled the body . . . ," we may comfort ourselves that our dislike for the body stands within the mainstream of our culture's struggles and preoccupations. And we may be even further comforted to discover that the Greeks, too, shared this dualism and assumed that the whole issue of warfare between body and mind belonged to men even more than to women. "It is natural," they said, "and expedient for the soul to govern the body, the intellect the emotions, man the lower animals, and the male the female."[3]

Buddhist thought, which undertakes to reconcile so many of the opposites we take for granted, fails in this effort so far as the body is concerned. Although the sacred art in the Buddhist tradition idealizes the body, much of the training of the Buddhist monk reveals precisely the opposite attitude. In his book on Buddhism, Edward Conze returns frequently to this idea. "Again and again," he writes, the monk "is taught to view this material body as repulsive, disgusting, and most offensive." Indeed, the monks in both the Buddhist and Jain traditions are instructed to meditate upon the body's "Nine Apertures, from which filthy and repulsive substances flow unceasingly. . . ."[4]

In this respect, the Buddhist tradition is consistent with Christian attitudes towards the body. Like the Christian, the Buddhist is not expected to delight or to take pride in the body, but is taught to feel "shame and disgust."[5]

But it is not only the philosophers and the theologians who concern themselves with this imperative task of reviling the body. The poets, too, have much to say about this oldest cultural issue. And the famous lines from Andrew Marvell may help us to understand just how widespread and pervasive is this dislike for the body from which so many of us suffer. "O who shall from its dungeon raise/This soul enslaved so many ways/With bonds of bone. . . ."

Our own most recent psychological thought regards man precisely as the paradoxical creature, half-animal and half-symbolic, and torn long between these poles. Indeed, as we learn from Ernest Becker, "in recent times every psychologist who had done vital work has made this paradox the main problem of his thought: Otto Rank . . . more consistently and brilliantly than anyone else since Kierkegaard, Carl Jung, Erich Fromm, Rollo May, Ernest Schachtel, Abraham Maslow, Harold H. Searles, Norman O. Brown, Laura Perls, and others."[6]

Man, the paradoxical creature, afflicted with an inner division between the self that thinks, reflects upon the world, and is called the mind, and that part of the self which is in nature and is called the body. And Becker claims that we learn this paradox, this conflict between the two essential parts of oneself unavoidably and in our earliest childhood.

> Often the child deliberately soils himself or continues to wet the bed, to protest against the imposition of artificial symbolic rules; he seems to be saying that the body is his primary reality and that he wants to remain in the simpler physical Eden and not be thrown out into the world of "right and wrong" . . . so we see that the two dimensions of human existence—the body and the self—can never be reconciled seamlessly.[7]

Let us for the moment follow this train of thought without necessarily endorsing it. Women, faced with a form of serious suffering over our bodies, must understand this issue in the most comprehensive and significant way. In our suffering over the size of our flesh we have been enacting an ancient quandary worthy of serious consideration and we should allow ourselves the dignity we deserve because of this. Correctly understood, our obsession is the stuff of which philosophy is made.

We are looking at the experience of the body that is common to children of both sexes and we are asking ourselves to understand the child's first sense of alienation from the body. For this problem, which is the principal issue in our obsession, may well have entered our lives when we were children. When we were learning, for instance, how much slower and more painstaking the body is than thought—a lesson repeated daily when, for example, the self-evidence of tying a pair of shoes became a frustrating and impossible task for the fingers. Somehow, in spite of the mind's clearly seeing how the shoe was tied, the fingers could not perform the task. Thus the body, stubborn or slow, requiring endless practice and repetition before it can even begin to approach the accomplishment of the simplest task, frustrates thought, calls into question the mind's sense of its own power, enrages the mind that cannot, for all its understanding, accomplish the tying of the shoe without the body. The body awakens in us a knowledge of our impotence, our inability to master the external world.

There were, of course, earlier problems with the body—the

way it hurt when it was not fed, when it grew cold and could not pull up its own covers, or when it was stuck by a pin that it could not remove from its own flesh and which no amount of thinking or imagining could remove. This pain, terrible in its own right, also forges the first link in our dependency upon others. We need them to bring us relief. It is the body that has made us vulnerable in this way. Reason, surely, to hate it.

But now we learn further that this vulnerability of our body places us within the sphere of another's power. Whether she comes to our aid and succors us in our distress becomes a matter of her determining, not to be accomplished by our will. But we had been imagining that if we thought of the coming of someone, she came; that our merest shriek had power to command the movements of others, or even that others were called by our unexpressed states of urgency and distress. We woke, felt fear, and even before we cried out, someone was there, lifting, warming, comforting us. Now, in the time that elapses between the cry and the answer to the cry, we learn through the body's unattended need the full measure of the mind's inability to command the obedience of the world.

Once we had imagined that if we imagined milk, this imaginary milk was sufficient to satisfy our needs. We made no distinction, in the youthfulness of our minds, between this milk in fantasy here within the mind, and that milk on our lips, outside there on the body. And now we know through the calling of hunger that is not instantly met how feeble is this power of the mind to satisfy the body's urgency. And for this knowledge, too, we blame the body.

And then, as Becker has seen, later on there is the learning of the necessity to govern the body. If we wish to be loved, praised, and awarded, and if we wish our parents to care for us, and if we wish to grow into girls and boys like our older brothers and sisters, we shall have to learn to master the excitements and eliminations of this body, keeping our hands strictly away from certain pleasurable parts and making certain some functions are performed in particular places, getting to the toilet on time and not being too interested in what the body does there, learning not to like the smell of what it creates and expels from itself and certainly not to touch it. But we fail in this again and again, touching, smelling, becoming fascinated, making our parents and older sisters angry at us and scornful, and trying again to conquer the body, and again giving way to its curious addiction to its own desires. For, yes, the body's stubborn insistence upon its pleasures makes us hate the body.

Then, if these are not yet reasons enough, there is always the fact that the body dies and takes us with it. We imagine heaven and the soul's continuance after death, the flight upward of winged creatures beyond the body's corruption, and yet even in our imaginings we invent a hell in which the body turns endlessly in its torments, pierced and roasted and deprived, endlessly spinning on a wheel of fire, pushing boulders up hills, and they roll down again, and there is fruit and it draws itself beyond our reach, and there is water that recedes when we stoop to sip it; and our own tears, brought on by the frustration of the body, burn our flesh like molten lead. For we are unable to imagine eternity without a body; unable to imagine this body without its vulnerability or to conceive of this body without imagining the suffering it makes for us.

So we behold the learning common to both women and men of reasons to dislike the body. There is no doubt, we say, that women and men share in what seems to be an unavoidable and universal condition.

And yet, something is missing in this account. For the fact remains that in this culture today, the most widespread expression of this alienation from the body occurs in the obsession with weight and dieting that afflicts millions of women. Men diet, too, they gain weight, there are certainly fat men in the world, and there are some men who lose so much weight they, too, are in danger of starving themselves to death. But it is women who constitute 95 percent of the people feeling sufficient despair with their bodies to enroll them in a formal program of weight reduction. Pick up the telephone and dial any diet organization in this country, ask them what percentage of their membership is female, and you will hear at first a tone of bewilderment that the question even needs to be asked. Then, the voice on the other end of the telephone will assure you that "most" of its membership is female, or "a lot," or "almost all of them." If you insist and ask for an actual number, you will discover, as I have, that it is 95 percent. You will find this to be the case, not with one or two diet organizations, but with all you are able to contact, all over the country. In spite of the fact that we have a common childhood experience in the learning of dislike for the body, men grow into adulthood without feeling an obsessive need to make the body smaller than it has been made by nature. Indeed, far from it. A man lifting weights, stripped to the waist in public, in full view of an admiring audience at the beach, is revealing a pride in his body. He is there to demonstrate his ability to expand, enlarge, and make it powerful, to increase the realm of the body precisely through the exercise of discipline and will. But women practice their obsession with the body in private. Alone, with despair, we glance into the mirror and down at the scale, hopeful and anguished in our quest for the body's reduction.

There are even more telling indications that women suffer more from living in the body than do men. For that precisely is the meaning of the fact that in this culture women regard themselves as fat if they are fifteen or twenty pounds overweight, while men do not enter these lists of despair until they are thirty-five pounds above the national average.[8] Of those 5,000 people each year who have their intestines removed in order to help themselves in their struggle to lose weight, 80 percent are women.[9] And finally, there is in this country a condition known as bulmarexia, in which periods of extreme eating are followed by self-induced vomiting. No one will be astonished to learn that almost every single human being troubled by this condition is a woman.[10]

Apparently, in this oldest struggle of mind against body, it is we, the women, who are driven to take it to its furthest extreme. And no one, through all the two thousand years of speculation about the mind/body division and warfare, has prepared us to understand why this might be so.

Not that opportunities for this understanding have been lacking, either. One would imagine, for instance, that the self-starvation of adolescent girls would offer students of the anorexic condition a wonderful opportunity to speculate about the connection between alienation from the body and the fact of being female. Anorexia is, after all, a condition in which mind struggles against body. It is also a distinctively woman's condition. No less than 90 percent of the people suffering from anorexia are female. But knowing this, we would, of course, expect that the most recent writers on anorexia would wonder about the relationship between the will to starve the body and the fact of being a woman. Aside, however, from Margaret Atwood, who is a novelist, almost no one does. The scientists, the psychologists, the family therapists all seem to be keeping a steady silence here. It is this fact which causes Sandra Gilbert (who is a literary historian) to ask this series of provocative questions:

> Why are 90 percent of anorexics female? Why don't most writers about anorexia nervosa explain why 90 percent of anorexics are female? Why has anorexia nervosa suddenly surfaced as the subject of so much popular speculation? . . . Although a number of books and articles I've read on this subject are useful and interesting, none makes the slightest attempt to answer any of these questions. . . . It is surprising, even puzzling, that none of these scientists attempts seriously to explore the evidently crucial relationship between anorexia nervosa and femaleness.[11]

There is serious indication in the psychological literature itself that anorexia nervosa reflects a girl's problem living, not merely in the body, but in a woman's body. Thus, Hilde Bruch writes of an adolescent girl suffering from anorexia: "It became apparent that part of her fight against gaining was her antagonism toward menstruation. Even though she had been menstruating for several years, she had never accepted it as a natural function."[12]

Of these girls in general she goes on to say: "They act as if no one had ever told them that developing curves and a certain roundness is a part of normal puberty." However, it is precisely at the moment they are about to develop into womanhood that these girls are seized by the anorexic longing. "Normal development and changes are interpreted as 'fatness,'" Hilde Bruch says. And this is surely the most revealing statement anyone can make. "Many have said that anorexics are expressing a fear of adulthood. They are actually afraid of becoming teenagers."

But here we may wish to disagree vehemently, and to wonder why Hilde Bruch infers, but does not make a direct connection between anorexia and a fear of being a woman. For it seems evident that anorexics are afraid of becoming, not adults, not teenagers, but women.

There is, in fact, a great deal of evidence for this in what anorexics say about themselves. Hilde Bruch has observed and recorded it and for this she is to be admired beyond most other students of the condition. But it is we who will have to take her observations on to the next level of generalization.

"From childhood on she felt it was not 'nice' to look like a woman, that her tissues would bulge, that the female body was not beautiful." Indeed, this attitude towards the female body becomes the litany of the anorexic quest. "There are people with flat stomachs," says an anorexic girl. "That is what I'm striving for. But I'm afraid I'm not built that way. My stomach is my Achilles' heel. I'm stuck with it and forced to admit something I've denied so far, that it is an inevitable fate." In the mind of these afflicted girls the female body becomes an inevitable fate—an unavoidable disaster. This is the characteristic vision of anorexia. "As long as it was below seventy pounds, she would without hesitation lift her nightgown to demonstrate to anyone that she was well-covered, that she really was fat, that there was nothing wrong with her body . . . as the weight increased and the slightest curves became noticeable, she became very modest, even prudish . . . now that she was voluptuous (weighing seventy-five pounds), she started to feel like a woman and wanted to keep her body private."

Inevitably, one of the girls, more conscious than the rest, will speak directly what is implicit in all the others. "I have a deep fear," says this girl, "of having a womanly body, round and fully developed."

What we have just heard is an astonishing insight, perhaps the most essential comment that can be made about the will to diet. And it can make us reflect that when a girl is afraid to develop a woman's body, the conflict she feels means more than even a struggle between mind and body. Anorexia nervosa now suggests that our tempestuous warfare against our bodies involves no less than a woman's identity as a woman.

6. SISTERS

> He is aware of a growing obsession with [her]. He would like to take a bite out of her. Purely an aesthetic consumption. He wants her to come across, to fork it over, to give him herself, the part, that is, which no one else has.
>
> —Ellen Schwamm

> If you are a mother you must let yourself be eaten, you must share yourself out at the feast. —Geza Roheim

> It is in great part the anxiety of being a woman that devastates the feminine body. —Simone de Beauvoir

"SHE LOOKED AROUND the room at all the women there, at the mouths opening and shutting, to talk or to eat . . . they all wore dresses for the mature figure. They were ripe, some rapidly becoming overripe, some already beginning to shrivel. . . . She examined the women's bodies with interest, critically . . . she could see the roll of fat pushed up across Mrs. Gundridge's back by the top of her corset, the ham-like bulge of thigh, the creases around the neck, the large porous cheeks; the blotch of varicose veins glimpsed at the back of one plump crossed leg, the way her jowls jellied when she chewed. . . ."

The young woman who is looking with such horrified fascination at the bodies of other women is Marian MacAlpin, the heroine of Margaret Atwood's novel, *Edible Woman.* [1] She is the typical "good" girl of our time, engaged to a "suitable" man whom she does not like, living with an excessively fatuous roommate with whom she has nothing in common, and going dutifully each day to a job that is perfectly meaningless to her. She moves along from one event to the next as if determined to fulfill all the conventional requirements of a young woman. She is eager to please, self-effacing, submissive, and eventually anorexic. Thus her body will have to express whatever uneasiness she feels about her life. This behavior on her body's part irritates her, of course. But the body will have its way. Reason, accusation, temptation, and even force only strengthen its resolution to refuse food. And Marian is finally reduced to the "forlorn hope that her body might change its mind." The body, however, does not change its mind. Having begun with steak, it eventually refuses soft-boiled egg and finally balks at even the innocent carrot, crying out for mercy from Marian's salad.

Marian is severely alienated from her body. She is also alienated from her emotional life. But she has no idea that her refusal of food is a significant emotional statement. To the reader, however, it becomes increasingly clear that Marian's body is constantly driven to confess feelings Marian herself disowns. Thus, when she is having a drink with the man who will shortly become her fiancé, she begins to stare at the reflections in the polished table at which they are sitting. "After a while," she says, "I noticed with mild curiosity that a large drop of something wet had materialized on the table near my hand. I poked it with my finger and smudged it around a little before I realized with horror that it was a tear. I must be crying then."

Needless to say, Marian is puzzled by her behavior and before long the narrative voice of the novel shifts from the first to the third person in order to record her increasing distance from knowledge of herself. To us, however, it is growing more and more apparent that both the body and the feelings of this woman have gained autonomy from her conscious intentions and that they will continue to behave in an erratic manner until she acknowledges and integrates them.

Marian, however, is on a wisdom journey. Her illness will one day be overcome and therefore what she sees and experiences along the way frequently takes on an astonishing depth of perception. Thus, at the Christmas office party, Marian experiences a revelation. Appearances are stripped away and she begins to see the problems with a woman's identity in this culture.

> Here, sitting like any other group of women at an afternoon feast, they no longer had the varnish of officialdom that separated them, during regular office hours, from the vast anonymous ocean of housewives whose minds they were employed to explore. They could have been wearing housecoats and curlers.[2]

Reading this passage, we begin to get our first inkling of what is troubling Marian about her own, female body, and making her wish to starve it, so that it loses all capacity to remind her that she, too, is a woman. For, in spite of the fact that she and her co-workers are employed in responsible jobs, there is no more essential meaning or satisfaction in their work than in the routine life of a housewife. Marian is discovering that women in this culture are deprived of a meaningful and authentic identity.

This might, of course, be a liberating moment for Marian. Inspired by this insight, she might stand up from her desk and walk out on her job. She might even break off her relationship with her boyfriend. But she remains seated and instead continues to muse. And now, what she muses upon offers us an essential insight into the workings of her illness. For it is at this moment that the ham-like bulge of Mrs. Gundridge's thigh makes its impression upon Marian. And there comes upon her now the full horror of life in the body.

"What peculiar creatures they were," Marian now thinks of these women who are celebrating Christmas with her: "taking things in, giving them out, chewing, words, potato chips, burps, grease, hair, babies, milk, excrement, cookies, vomit, coffee, tomato juice, blood, tea, sweat, liquor, tears, and garbage. . . ."

This horror of a fleshly existence shorn of meaning is the very essence of the anorexic vision. It may well be the typical vision of our time. Sooner or later, if we allow it to influence us without examining its implications, we, too, shall be wishing to get out of this flesh that carries us about through the world, taking things in, giving them out, involving itself in the whole cycle of ripening and shriveling, of growing mature. For it is precisely the life cycle itself Marian has been pondering in her terrified and stricken way. "You were green," she reflects, "and then you ripened; became mature. Dresses for the mature figure. In other words, fat."

In the equation Marian constructs, fat stands for maturity and maturity implies a meaningless existence. And yet, it is clearly not the large size of these women, or their maturity, or their pleasure in eating, or the act of eating itself, which should be blamed for what has happened in their lives. Marian has just accepted the conventional explanations of her culture, which hold that a woman's fat body is responsible for everything that is lacking in her life. Her moment of vision has collapsed into a conventional blaming of the flesh.

But this false blaming of the body is part of Marian's illness. It is part also of her inability to liberate herself from the impoverished identity that is troubling her. Because she is a compliant girl she cannot manage to free herself from her fiancé or refuse to go to her job. But she can refuse to let her body mature and make her a woman like the women she observes. By turning back the biological clock she hopes to avoid the adaptations which our culture requires of women. That is the real meaning of her inability to eat.

There are, however, consequences in store for Marian. Indeed, one immediate result of her alienation from her body is the fact that she is severely alienated from nature as she struggles to place herself outside the life process that brings her to maturity. Thus, her unexamined protest involves her in a tragic estrangement from the organic cycle that is potentially a source of woman's power.

For the anorexic girl, as for many women who diet, this alienation from nature is the price we pay for our inability to speak directly and with full self-knowledge our uneasiness about our female identity, as it is offered to us by our culture. We cannot grow ripe, we cannot mature, we never appreciate the power of our kinship with nature, we fail to wonder that our menstrual cycle is influenced by the moon and that our seasons of psychic and emotional life belong as much to the cosmos as the ocean's tides. We, whose bodies know how to conceive and create life, whose breasts know how to bring forth food from themselves, despise these bodies that possess the very power the world's great religions regard as divine. Thus, we begin to appreciate how much we are losing in this warfare against the body—how dangerously we are being pitted against our authentic identity as women.

Marian, it is true, finally overcomes this alienation from woman's natural power. She suceeds finally in being honest with herself about what she is feeling. And through this honesty she rediscovers a knowledge of ancient practices and invents all over again the lost mythology in the making of food. She decides to bake a cake. But this is no ordinary cake Marian has hit upon for the purpose of liberating herself from the self-effacing person she has been. This is a cake shaped in the figure of a woman.

> The cake looked peculiar with only a mouth and no hair or eyes. She rinsed out the cake decorator and filled it with chocolate icing. She drew a nose, and two large eyes, to which she appended many eyelashes and two eyebrows. . . . For emphasis she made a line demarcating one leg from the other, and similar lines to separate the arms from the body.[3]

This cake Marian now offers to her fiancé, as an expression of her fully conscious awareness that he (and the conventional society for which he stands) have been trying to eat her up. "You've been trying to destroy me, haven't you?" she asks him. "You've been trying to assimilate me. But I've made you a substitute, something you'll like much better."

Her boyfriend, however, does not accept this substitute. He cannot acknowledge the meaning of what is being enacted here. He refuses to understand that in his relationship with Marian he has been trying to destroy all the elemental hungers and assertions of which she is capable as a female being. His eyes widen in alarm when he is offered this cake. Unnerved, he stares from the cake to Marian and back again. Then, he rapidly takes leave of her.

And now, of course, Marian's hunger returns. She no longer has to speak mutely through her body and the suppression of her appetites to express all that has been troubling her about her identity as a woman. She is free to hunger and to feel. It is she now who must devour the cake. It is the moment for an exquisite transposition of meaning.

For Marian, as she begins to chew and swallow, is symbolically reclaiming her hunger and her right to hunger. By eating up this cake fetish of a woman's body she assimilates for the first time her own body and its feelings. It is re-enactment of the ritual feast, in which the eating of an animal's flesh, or a piece of cake shaped like a breast, signifies the coming together of human and divine, individual with collective, tribal ancestor with member of the tribe, human community with nature, or a woman with her own body and feelings. Marian has transcended the futile symbolism of anorexia and evolved instead the expressive symbolism of ritual.

Unfortunately, however, Marian is rare; few anorexic girls come upon this solution, which restored Marian to her feelings and her body, placed her back within nature, and reunited her with a spontaneous source of imaginative power, through which her need for a positive female identity can be spoken consciously. Most anorexic girls, if they do not find psychological help or feminist understanding, will continue to sacrifice nature, their bodies, their power, their health, and their well-being, perhaps for the rest of their lives.

Slenderness carries meanings. The slender girl in our culture is not the healthy antithesis of the pathological fat woman, but is in fact her sister—the kinship forged by the emotional attitudes that find expression through the body but remain otherwise mute, unknown, and unexamined.

This sisterhood between the gaunt and the obese becomes dramatically apparent when we place next to Marian another heroine of Margaret Atwood's who also has a distinctive relationship to food. But this young woman, known as Lady Oracle, finds that she never wishes to stop eating. Taken together, the slender, self-effacing Marian and the fat, rebellious Lady Oracle form the poles that define our position as women in contemporary culture today, so far as the use of our body to express meaning is concerned. For just as Marian in her refusal of food has instructed us in the hidden intentionality of anorexia, Lady Oracle through her gluttony lets us in on the secret strategy of being fat.

Indeed, Lady Oracle has glimpsed the fact that her mother has taken up a decidedly proprietary interest in her daughter's body —that she hopes to make her daughter into an object that will reflect glory upon the mother. "If she'd ever gone out and done it," says Lady Oracle, "she wouldn't have seen me as a reproach to her, the embodiment of her own failure and depression, a huge endless cloud of inchoate matter which refused to be shaped into anything for which she could get a prize."[4] Understandably enough, the daughter is outraged by her mother's intervention in her life and she determines to defeat her mother's intention to make her into a socially acceptable product. Thus, by the age of thirteen, the daughter is "eating steadily, doggedly, stubbornly," anything she can get. And she tells us that "the war between myself and my mother was on in earnest; the disputed territory was my body."

The fatness of this woman is a protest; in it we are enabled to read many kinds of hostility and a great deal of emotional distress. Lady Oracle talks about eating from panic and from a need to defy her mother; she grows fat in order to assert her own power to refuse to let her mother make her over in "her image, thin and beautiful." She is fat to protect herself against male sexual aggression. "Although my mother had warned me about bad men in the ravine, by the time I reached puberty her warnings rung hollow. She clearly didn't believe I would ever be molested, and neither did I. It would have been like molesting a giant basketball and secretly, though I treasured images of myself exuding melting femininity and soft surrender, I knew I would be able to squash any potential molester against a wall merely by breathing out."[5] And she is fat finally in order to shame and embarrass her mother socially. "I no longer attended my mother's dinner parties; she was tired of having a teenaged daughter who looked like a beluga whale and never opened her mouth except to put something into it. I cluttered up her hostess act."

Margaret Atwood is a brilliant writer and she has, in these two novels, glimpsed the vital connection between our nutritional malaise and our problems being a woman in this culture. Taken together, these books bear witness to the fact that the anorexic girl and the obese woman have a great deal in common. An unexpressed hostility, fear of sexuality, an uneasiness about what is expected of women in this culture, prompt both of them to take up their distinctive attitude towards food. Both are alienated from the body, and their natural power as women; both are, at least in the beginning, unable to express their emotional condition articulately and directly. Both use the body for the purposes of such expression. There is panic and self-hatred in both of them.

There are two other women who can help us to understand the metaphorical meanings of a woman's body, and we can find them in Margaret Laurence's wonderful novel *The Fire-Dwellers.* As it happens, one of these women is like many of us in her feeling about the body. She wakes up in the morning, catches a glimpse of herself in the mirror and thinks: "Everything would be all right if only I was better educated. . . . Or if I were beautiful. Okay, that's asking too much. Let's say if I took off ten or so pounds." This thought captivates her and her mind continues to play with it. Now she addresses herself. "Listen, Stacey," she says, "at thirty-nine, after four kids, you can't expect to look like a sylph." And then she answers this truth with the following reflection: "Maybe not, but for hips like mine there's no excuse." But now, when the pain of this observation becomes unbearable, she resorts to that favorite fantasy among large women. "I wish," she says, "I lived in some country where broad-beamed women were fashionable."[6]

The other woman in this story lives next door to Stacey and she, whose name is Tess, embodies everything our culture desires for a woman. She is tall and slender; even in a housecoat she looks "as though ready to receive the Peruvian ambassador." Already, at an early hour of the morning, her hair is done in a "flawless French Roll." She has no problem controlling her appetite, lives on cottage cheese and pineapple, and is so beautiful that her own husband, as he later confesses, has never been able to know her, so incredible has it seemed to him that she would marry him at all. Even Stacey, whose heart is as large at least as her hips, could see no suffering in Tess, so blinded was she by the glamour.

Stacey and Tess. The one with nonexistent hips, with wonderful taste in clothes, with the high-pitched girlish voice, which remains uncertain in spite of Tess' accomplishment in becoming everything we all envy in this culture. The other with hips too large, a large woman who drinks too much, who longs to have love affairs, who gets drunk at her husband's office party, who takes a lover, who cannot stay on her diet, who one day puts on shamrock velvet pants, a petunia purple blouse, cheap gilt high-heeled sandals, and goes prancing and squirming and jiggling with a glass of gin in her hand in the basement of her house. Tess and Stacey. The large woman so filled with the force of sensuality and natural power it cannot possibly be contained by the conventional role of housewife and mother, but spills out and transforms every relationship and draws people to her and sustains life. The slender woman so filled with despair she one day swallows a bottle of rye with enough sleeping pills to almost kill her.

It is at this point that we realize a remarkable transformation of vision has been taking place in this novel. For, as we have come to love and admire Stacey, it begins to seem to us that her body is changed before our eyes, so that this face, which is "heavier than once," these hips and ass, which are bigger than she would like, have begun finally to seem beautiful as they take on the meaning of the woman's emotional amplitude.

But the transformation works in the opposite direction as well, for we discover a ravaging hunger in the slenderness of Tess, who is found one day holding Stacey's youngest daughter in a chair, pressing her hands against the child's shoulders as the little girl squirms and tries to get away, while Tess forces her to look into a fishbowl where one fish is devouring another. In this moment, the glamour of Tess, with her well-coiffed hair, transposes itself into the image of a death's-head.

As the story ends, Stacey and Tess reverse their symbolic positions. The beauty of Tess has been stripped away, to reveal desperation, an eerie fascination with the natural life, with the organic cycle, with appetite and with the devouring aspects of self she has created by disowning her own, natural hunger. And the large-hipped Stacey, with her unruly hair, has been transformed into an embodiment of the life force, of woman's power according to nature. Tess lies in the hospital, recovering from the effort to destroy herself, in which she has been engaged for years. Stacey lies awake in bed, still planning to go on a diet, but knowing now that she will not be able to keep herself from growing larger and larger. For she is a woman who has discovered that one day, "given another forty years," she may eventually "mutate into a matriarch."

7. THE MATRIARCH

> We are heavy with bodies. If men bore children, we imagine, they would burst from their heads, not their asses, and be fully grown, and dressed, and godlike, with no need to eat, no substance pouring from their substance. But we are mothers. . . .
> —Susan Griffin

> Naturally, I here mean Bachofen. This gentle, corpulent Basel patrician, with the wonderfully rounded child's mouth . . . and an almost unbelievable understanding, in his profound, inner loneliness, discovered the female era at the lower seam of history, with its sacerdotal, political, and economic female dominion.
> —Helen Diner

> Wherever the goddess is superior to the god, and ancestresses more reverently worshipped than ancestors, there is nearly always a mother-kin structure.
> —Sir James Frazer

THE TRANSFORMATION we have just witnessed would be possible for us, too, if we were able to remember. Ancient, forgotten, dimly present at the edge of consciousness, the image of the matriarch carries with it a sense of what a large woman, large in body and appetite, large in her longing for life, in her capacity to create, to take pleasure and to feed her hungers, might mean.

And so it will profit us to begin the process of remembering, struggling consciously to acquire an imagery which speaks against the limitations of our contemporary vision of a woman's body. We are in search of vision that will help us to live comfortably within our own bodies, an imagery that is part of our effort to reclaim our bodies from a culture that has alienated them, along with so many other sources of our power and pleasure. Images of large women that can make us proud.

For me, the process of remembering begins with a woman I have observed over the years, fascinated by the periodic changes in the size of her body. At my daughter's school, in a neighborhood gourmet food store, at the opera, or at the opening of an art exhibit, I would often catch sight of a vaguely familiar stranger, who upon closer scrutiny would turn out to be my acquaintance, always at first unrecognizable in her new disguise, sometimes in a leather suit, her hair cut short, her body gaunt and angular—that year she was studying to become a lawyer; at other times, plump and curly-haired, wearing long skirts and loose blouses, grinding her own whole wheat flour at home and baking extraordinary concoctions for the school's spring festival. But then, one day, this woman grew very fat. At the same time, she was deeply absorbed in her newest enthusiasm—working day and night as a sculptor. Only now something was different than it had been before. She neglected her home, she didn't prepare meals anymore, she refused to shop. Her husband, a physician, was certain all this was an expression of her hostility toward him and the children. And therefore, when she began to be successful, when several small galleries started to exhibit her work, he was irritated at first. Later, he became more accepting of it and finally now, he assured me, proud.

As for the woman herself, when I saw her at the opening of her show, she looked better to me than I'd ever seen her before. This new, fat body of hers seemed positively radiant with the pride and power of her accomplishment. She was standing at the center of the room a glass of champagne in her hand. She was huge now, there could be no doubt of it. And I continued to be surprised that I found her more appealing than before. There she was, a distinctly massive figure, with broad hips, large breasts, standing with her legs apart, in a definite posture of self-assertion. And she was laughing, a laugh such as I'd never heard from her before—husky, sensual, and provocative. Around her, in the room, were equally massive figures and shapes, sometimes the torsos of huge women, sometimes a form that suggested a thigh, a breast, an immense, rounded belly. Among these figures I now wandered entranced, as much by the way the sculptor had fashioned her own image in these diverse forms, as by the fact that they had become for me a moment of illumination. Through them, for the first time in my life, I was coming to understand how the large size of a woman might stand for more than a dislike for the self; might represent an assertion of power, of eros, of the rights and dignities of flesh. I was captivated by this vision; through it, I sensed, something old and forgotten was coming back to me. I wrote a letter of appreciation to this woman and a few days later she called me.

"I know I should feel ashamed of myself," she said. "And often I do. I eat too much, I drink too much, I talk too loud, I keep a messy house. But I have moments. After I've been at work. I get undressed, I look in the mirror. I realize it's my own body I've been modeling all day. Rings of flesh, massive plains, mountainous plateaus of flesh. Suddenly, I'm in a glory of fleshly existence. I see power in it, in my own body, fertility, abundance. A large, unrestricted sense of life. I dream about huge women. They've always been very appealing to me. And so I wake up thinking, why shouldn't I be one of them? I can't say I'm ever actually proud of the way I look when I go out in public. But I get intimations of pride. Then, if I think about Barry, the way he's ashamed to introduce me to his friends, I think, the hell with him. I'm sick of whittling myself down to size. I'm a mountain of a woman, he thinks? Well, if he's so much of a man, let him climb me."

All this happened some years ago; since then, I've lost track of my acquaintance, my daughter has moved on to another school, we have moved away from San Francisco. Every so often I scan the art news, wondering if I can catch sight of those monumental women who initiated me into a new way of looking at a woman's body. But I have not seen mention of them again. Consequently, I don't know whether the enthusiasm of the sculptor lasted, whether she is still carving her massive forms, still carrying about in her own body this radical vision of the flesh. But now, recalling her, I see her as a lonely, early pioneer, tearing herself bodily out of her husband's culture, where she was expected to be slender and elegant, demure and refined, with a clean house, regular meals on the table, a polite and modulated form of talk.

Recently, I came across an ancient personality who reminded me of this sculptor, not so much because of her large size, as for a quality of spirit and personality she had in common with my friend. I was reading a description of Baubo, who was closely associated with Aphrodite, and who belonged to women more than she did to men. As Nor Hall describes her, "she danced and sang before Demeter, told obscene (filthy or piggy) stories, and gave birth to laughter—specifically 'belly laughs.' "[1]

That, I think, is a disturbing and astonishing description, reminding us that there were peoples and places, whole cultures where women were permitted more than our culture allows. The women of these early times were larger, both in their bodies and in the range of qualities permitted to them. Reading of these times we learn of old forms of goddess worship, of how Venus-Aphrodite asks "to be praised with "animal" lovemaking. Cats and other animals lie with exposed parts like the pig-riding Baubo, who comes with legs wide-spread carrying a ladder."[2] This is the "ladder-of-the-soul," and it reminds us that the initiate can go up and down, back and forth, between the "mud realm of Baubo . . . to the transcendant starry heaven of Venus." And this, indeed, is precisely what I saw years ago, without understanding it, as I looked at the sculptor on the opening day of her exhibit. For it was precisely this profound reconciliation of opposites that was made evident for me by the sight of a fat woman who had become an artist. Her art inseparable from the celebration of fatness. The power of this art, when it began to operate within the woman herself, awakening a love for food, a willingness to eat and indulge herself, and to take pleasure in her body.

And so we begin to wonder, whether something of this, a wisp, a memory, speaks to us still in the body of a fat woman and calls us back to the body, back to our sensuality, back to our appetite, back to our power. For indeed, this knowledge of the power of woman must once have been the very essence of goddess worship. Then, the body of a large woman, sculpted over and over again, through countless prehistoric cultures, stood for this overcoming of separations, for the reconciliation of mud and heaven, spirit and flesh, individual and collective, human and divine.

What a highly subversive and seductive note rings from these descriptions of the body of the goddess.

> . . . the matriarchal peoples feel the unity of all life, the harmony of the universe, which they have not yet out-grown . . . They yearn more fervently for higher consolation, in the phenomena of natural life, and they relate this consolation to the generative womb, to conceiving, sheltering, nurturing mother love. No era has attached so much importance to outward form, *to the sanctity of the body.* [3]

But how amazing this must seem when placed alongside our own contemporary sense of these things, the body of the women in the cafeteria, as seen through the eyes of our own anorexic heroine—the ham-like thighs, the porous cheeks, the jowls jellied, the roll of fat above the corset.

Or compare this anorexic vision with these descriptions of the goddess by Nor Hall, who remembers the past. "Bedrock of being," she calls this sculpture of the goddess, "full and immobile, a mountain of a woman asleep with her ear to the ground."[4] And again: "The mother whose breasts never run dry . . . resting on great rounds . . . a fertility object. The subject is life abundant, radiating from her mid-region."[5]

Who in our time would think to describe a fat woman in these terms? Perceiving in her these qualities of fundamental, bedrock existence, sensual pleasures, nurturant force, the dance and the laughter which equally are of the earth and sky? What fat woman of our day could possibly perceive her body through this vision, which has never heard of the horror of the body, the effort to subdue or control it, or make it less than nature has intended it to be? In our time the fat woman looks at herself as Lady Oracle does; nothing else seems possible. "I didn't usually look at my body," says Lady Oracle, "in a mirror or in any other way . . . the whole thing was too overwhelming. There, staring me in the face, was my thigh. It was enormous, it was gross, it was like a diseased limb, the kind you see in pictures of jungle natives; it spread on forever . . . the flesh not green but bluish-white, with veins meandering across it like rivers."[6]

And yet, through all this horror which finally drives Lady Oracle to reduce her flesh, there peeps an old association—that ancient, forgotten memory of a time when the body of a woman was seen in glory like the body of the earth. "Sanctity of the body. Body inviolate, fused with the earth . . . this Mother is the hill itself. She is a mountainous mass of earth whose headdress must seem to graze the heavens from the perspective of the small creature who depends upon her for food and support."[7]

A fat woman carries in her body the evocative power of the matriarch. She may have become fat in order to spite her mother, she may have made herself fat to avoid her sexuality and convince herself that she is ugly, but even in this extreme condition the more basic, more primordial meaning of fatness is simultaneously present in the earth imagery she uses to describe herself. For we have two simultaneous, but highly divergent responses to our own bodies—one which is conditioned by our culture and makes us see the large size of our flesh as hideous and unattractive; the other which arises spontaneously from an archetypal source, reversing the cultural values and showing us the redemptive possibilities in our own large size.

It frequently happens that when the dominant culture loses a vision or actively suppresses it, this lost knowledge arises again among those excluded from that culture. Thus, if we wish to discover other meanings in the large size of a woman, we should look at works in which it is women who are fashioning the portraits of women. There, we can see the body portrayed without hatred, without fear of its girth, without horror at its rolls of flesh.

Looking, for instance, at the photograph of Princess Eugène Murat by Berenice Abbot,[8] we see a large, a fat woman who is decidedly elegant, sitting with one elbow resting on the arm of her chair. Monumentally, without apology for herself, she sits with one hand holding a cigarette, a look in her eyes which is tough, hard, a challenge but not a provocation, a willingness to measure herself, as she is, against all the tough hard meanness of the world. Her large size speaks power, from the body of a woman accustomed to being obliged. There is not the slightest possibility we would be tempted to laugh at this woman, to mock her for her obesity, to make of her a figure of fun. This woman is used to command and she commands respect.

Or there is that portrait of an old woman by Dorothea Lange[9] standing in the Berryessa Valley of California, in a field of poppies, holding out her hand. She is a woman large and full with nurturance, her simple print dress tied at the waist, shaping her into a pear, so that we see her as part of the field in which she stands, as much a part of nature as the poppies. It is a wonderful portrait of an old woman who can offer home without giving too much of herself; there is a simple pride visible in every line of the face, as in the low, rounded bosoms, the ample stomach rising to support them, an intelligence that speaks equally from the body and the eyes.

"The Hurricane," by Germaine Richier, the personifying figure of a large woman who seems to be listening to her own pulse and heartbeat, her own rhythm. And so she stands with a large, rounded belly and large waist, with that look of supreme self-acceptance in her face, as one who "accepts that her center of gravity is herself."[10]

The mother and child by Paula Modersohn-Becker, sleeping together, curled toward one another in an enveloping, sensuous curve, the woman all roundness, of large belly and hips and legs and breasts, casting even a round shadow, as the child curls into this body it would be blasphemy to call obese, so powerfully does it stand for mothering.[11]

What is apparent here, through all the diversity of styles and media and forms, is the fact that these large women inspire no revulsion and feel none for themselves; in these big bodies there is not the slightest trace of self-hatred or shame, suppressed rage or hostility, nothing the least bit pathological, neither hatred for the mother nor extreme antagonism for the self; there is no evidence of emotional distress which drives the woman to eat more than she desires for her pleasure; there is no alienation from the flesh, so that it appears grotesque, either to the beholder, or to the woman-spirit it carries, which is here sensitive and intelligent, masterful, and proud. We call up the words pride and grace to describe these women in their large bodies; we speak of warmth and nurturance, of the dignity of flesh, its "heavy dignity, its primitive strength,"[12] its "monumental massiveness," for we know that these are women as women regard them, with a vision that poses a radical critique to this culture with its tyranny of slenderness, its hatred for the flesh. A vision in which the spirit enters again through the body and is, in all its fullness and abundance, so gratefully embodied there.

"I've drawn a young mother with the child at her breast," Paula Modersohn-Becker wrote in her diary, "sitting in her smoke filled hut. . . . A sweet woman, a 'Karitas.' She was breast-feeding the large one-year-old bambino. And the four-year-old girl with the sulky eyes was snatching and grabbing at the breast until she got it. And the woman was giving her life and her youth and strength to the child in all simplicity, without realizing that she was a heroic figure."[13]

It is not only women who are capable of the reconciliation between spirit and body that is characteristic of the matriarchal vision. Men, too, would be capable of this redemptive vision if they were at peace with the natural side of themselves, which in this culture is associated with women. Then, indeed, we might expect that their expression of this accomplishment would take the form of paintings and sculptures of large, abundant women, who retain their subjectivity, their capacity to think and muse deeply, all the intelligence that is compatible with woman's power and sensual fulfillment. Indeed, whatever image the male painter and sculptor then shapes in his work, it will be an embodiment of his own feminine nature. Even when he uses a woman for a model, he will have created an image of his reconciliation with what is sensual and spiritual in himself.

It is this vision of reconciliation I see in the paintings of Renoir, particularly in the late work of this man who claimed that without the female body he would not have become a painter. According to Kenneth Clark, Renoir was a man of serene and "sunny temperament," and this fact is relevant when we consider that he is also one of the great masters of the female nude, creating those lovely, abundant girls who brought him his greatest popularity, but evolving also "a new race of women, massive, ruddy, unseductive but with the weight and unity of great sculpture."[14] It should come then as no surprise to us that this artist married a woman of large and generous proportions and painted her as *La Baigneuse blonde,* serene, contemplative, available to wisdom, her body evocative as fruit and powerful as the body of an ancient goddess. It seems evident that this artist was gifted with an absence of conflict about the physical side of existence. And so he painted women who become, then, more than women, who are able to embody that feminine side of life in which light plays over the sensual surface of things, dissolving contours, merging figure and ground, drowning everyone present in a celebration of undifferentiated oneness.

Instinctively we know that this affirmative vision requires the women this painter uses for his models to be as large as possible, so that the sheer magnitude of life's richness can be embodied in an expressive and representational form. Thus, the women in a Renoir canvas are huge; by our standards they are fat and they become, with their voluptuous abundance, portraits of life *(la vie),* dancing, bathing, forever in motion, life contemplative along the riverside, and one is drawn towards them through a force that is larger than the sexual, drawn down into this feminine side of existence, with its rounded forms and dappled surfaces, its rose tints and hues, which seem to stand for sensuality itself; for a woman's body flushing with pleasure at a supreme moment of sensual fulfillment, this hue which pervades his work and seems to fill it with the permission to delight in and lose oneself in a sensual existence.

For it is indeed love of the body we discover finally in the paintings of Renoir. These women are fecund, fertile, nubile, ripe, pregnant, abundant, ebullient, teeming, swelling. And the image of them opens out beyond the painting, into one's own affirmation of life, into one's longing for the half-fearful, half-joyous delirium of the painter, wandering the back streets of Montparnasse, intoxicated by the heat of the late hour, the smells of the blossoming fruit trees, the forbidden odor of the urinals, and of sugared almonds from the street vendor's stall.

8. THE BOUTIQUE

> It is now fashionable to be thin, but if it were fashionable to be fat, women would force-feed themselves like geese, just as girls in primitive societies used to stuff themselves because the fattest girl was the most beautiful. If the eighteen-inch waist should ever become fashionable again, women would suffer the tortures of tight lacing, convinced that though one dislocated one's kidneys, crushed one's liver, and turned green, beauty was worth it all. —Una Stannard

WELL THEN, why can't we manage to be proud of our large bodies? Why can't we altogether grasp the fact that there might be something of a positive nature in the very fact of fleshly existence? What, we say? Woman's abundance, her fullness of body, her potbelly and her fat ass and her big thighs regarded as beauty? Somehow it remains very hard for us to imagine women fashioning an ideal image for ourselves that required us to be grand and voluptuous. We can't quite conceive what it would be like to take back to ourselves the right to decide how our bodies should look, choosing an aesthetic according to health and nature, wishing our bodies to bear witness to our celebration of appetite, natural existence, and women's power.

And yet we do know that there were times, not so long ago, when women did not feel about their bodies the way we do. Then, a woman considered it a disaster if she stepped on the scale and found that she had lost weight. There once actually were women who had no respect for the anxieties of their physicians, who went ahead and caused their doctors to feel despair. These women would not lose weight because they did not wish to, and they did not wish to because their bodies seemed more beautiful to them when they were fat.

A physician in that day actually complained that it was fashion and aesthetic that interfered with prescribed weight-reducing programs.

> One must mention here that asethetic errors of a worldly nature to which all women submit, may make them want to stay obese for reasons of fashionable appearance. It is beyond a doubt that in order to have an impressive decollete each woman feels herself duty bound to be fat around the neck, over the clavicle and in her breasts. Now it happens that fat accumulates with greatest difficulty in these places and one can be sure, even without examining such a woman, that the abdomen and the hips, and the lower members are hopelessly fat. As to the treatment, one cannot obtain weight reduction of the abdomen without the woman sacrificing in her spirits the upper part of her body. To her it is a true sacrifice because she gives up what the world considers beautiful.[1]

That was in 1911. And the little parable tells us one thing quite clearly. If the standard of beauty that prevailed in Paris in 1911 were still in fashion in America of 1980, none of us would go home tonight after a large meal, and take laxatives, and run the risk of ruining our digestion, upsetting our electrolyte imbalance, and disturbing the natural condition of the flora of our intestine. If we were admired for having fat around the neck, as women were in 1911, and were permitted to have large abdomens and well-padded hips, tens of thousands of women would not kneel down next to the toilet tonight and put our fingers down our throat, and vomit.

From this simple fact we come to appreciate, all over again, the way an aesthetic ideal affects our lives with an extreme coercive power. Fashion lets us know what our culture expects us to be, or to become, or to struggle to become, in order to be acceptable to it, thereby exercising a devastating power over our lives on a daily basis. The image of women that appears in the advertisement of a daily newspaper has the power to damage a woman's health, destroy her sense of well-being, break her pride in herself, and subvert her ability to accept herself as a woman.

Thus, it is possible to study fashion the way one can study a work of art, so that it reflects significantly upon the issues and conflicts of its own day. The nude body of a woman, as we have seen, carries a tale that proves interesting beyond the boundaries of aesthetic speculation. Similarly, fashion, in the image it creates of woman, expresses itself on a variety of issues its makers would never imagine so deeply concerned them. By studying the face, the expression, the body, the gesture of the recurring images in our culture, we begin to read our culture's attitudes toward power in a woman, her sensual freedom, her right to joyfulness, subjectivity, and expressiveness through her body, her right to age, to grow mature in her body, to acquire authority, to bear this authority in the angle of her jaw, the settling back of her shoulders, the tilt of her head. If the pages of *Vogue* presented us with pictures of large women, their bodies muscular like those of athletes, their heads held high like those of a person of prestige and influence; if the pages of the daily newspaper showed women wearing clothes that emphasized the beauty of a powerful back, the strength of a large hip, hands and feet that were able to work and to accomplish, necks that were capable of carrying life's burden, or a softness, a fullness and abundance that seemed, like a ripening fruit, to stand for the abundance and fullness of life itself, there would not be six million women in this country today who had joined Weight Watchers to change the size of their bodies; eight thousand of us next week would not be moving through the doors of the diet salon, and the word bulmarexia might never have had to be created, in 1974, to describe our unique cultural disorder—a disease that includes simultaneously the symptoms of insatiable appetite (bulemia) and (anorexia) the rejection of food.[2]

But it is also true that the fashions we are speaking about have changed several times since 1911; we know that during the 1920s, women were binding their breasts and bobbing their hair and hoping to look like boys; and we remember that in 1960 Marilyn Monroe, when she made the film *Some Like It Hot,* was still permitted to be as large as a woman in a drawing by Modersohn-Becker. We who fell in love with her then and yearned as growing girls to look like her, seeing this film now, and the size of the woman who was our heroine, must marvel at what has happened to our very perception of beauty. For Monroe, if she were alive now, and still as grand and voluptuous as she was then, would today no doubt be considered fat. It is unlikely that today someone seeing her for the first time would be taken with jealousy because of the abundance in her body, the way Susan Strasberg was, the first time she saw her. "We were talking after the scene," says Strasberg, "when suddenly a stream of energy vitalized the stage. Heads began to turn and people stared as Marilyn Monroe undulated across the room in a dress so fitted she could barely move. I was instantly jealous of her, her *zaftig* body, her blondeness, the ease with which she commanded attention."[3]

But this zaftig body of Monroe, when it appears on a woman of our time, becomes a source of profound despair; it is measured, frowned upon, afflicted with starvation, hidden away, and taken finally into surgery, where for $2,500 the buttocks are reduced, and where for another $3,000 the thighs are made smaller, and where for yet more thousands of dollars the roundness of the belly is made flat. Because fashion dictates an extreme slenderness for women in our time, cosmetic surgeons become wealthy, they have offices with large Jacuzzi bathtubs for their own relaxation, staffs that include a full-time anesthesiologist, seven nurses, and operating rooms that open upon the "chandeliered conference/dining room that affords a view" of the operating table itself.[4] In our culture today, all this is taken so much for granted that the glossy, color pictures in a perfectly respectable magazine show us the office manager of the surgeon, whose success depends primarily on women's despair, quietly cutting into a melon, while behind her three doctors make an incision into their patient.

And so we make our way into the street life of our culture, hoping now to look again, with a new quality of perception, at the most commonplace expression of the conflicts and dilemmas that inspire literature and art, philosophy and psychological perceptions. But we are now not surprised to find that the conflict over the flesh is reflected here too, in this stamping ground of the anorexic heroine, whose picture is repeated on every page of the fashion magazine, and whose form is sculpted in the stylish mannequins of the store windows, and whose representative greets us, with a false smile, a secret disparagement, as we enter a clothing store, for it is clear that we enter without being able to conform—we will need a size nine or ten or maybe eleven; we will not do justice to the new, slender line, the tapering curve at the hip, the girdle-like constriction of the jeans. How often we have been filled with panic, catching a glimpse of ourselves, in all our unredeemed femininity, looking back with a frantic expression from the mirrors that reflect everything we are supposed to be —those girls who have succeeded where we have failed, those long-limbed mannequins who have become our omnipresent reminder, our reproach.

We enter the shop; it is called a boutique and it summons us because it is one of those hallowed places which were never really intended for the likes of us. On other occasions it may have been a wistful fantasy that brought us in here, seeing the redheaded plastic mannequin in the window, with her raffish scarf and tangled hair—a wild hope that our own unaccommodations to fashion might be accommodated here. And so we suck in our stomachs, straightening our shoulders as we take ourselves to the nearest rack. But in this shop the sizes seem to have been shrinking. The signs on the rack are bold and explicit—they wish to make it clear that here, in the showplace of our culture, some significant transformation has occurred. SIZE THREE? But what has happened to the sevens or the nines? The place is thick with ones and twos and there, shame-facedly in the far corner, is a rack of fives. They don't have size nine, the girl tells us, although we have not asked. "But don't you know," we want to say to her, "that there are over twenty-five million women in this country who wear size sixteen and over? That, if you want to know, is more than 30 percent of the women in this land.[5] And what of all the rest of us, uncounted, who are unable to adapt ourselves to these styles suited for adolescents? And what, if you come to that, do you make of the fact that the large size clothes are called, in the vernacular of the garment industry, 'women's sizes,' and just what, if you follow me, does that reveal about these gaunt garments hanging here? For surely, you see that they were not intended for a woman?" But, of course, we do not utter this frenzy of protest against the fashions. We have been too busy wondering how the girl guessed we wore size nine. Last year, she wouldn't have dared.

And so, we remind ourselves, it was not always like this; there were other times, and places, where woman in her abundance was a celebration. We recall scraps of song, pieces of literature that have always served to reassure us. And we repeat to ourselves, as we rush from the store, these words the young men used to sing in the Copper Belt of Rhodesia, this song of courtship. "Hullo Mama, the beautiful one, let us go to the town. You will be very fat, you girl, if you stay with me."[6] But does this comfort us? We need more support, we are besieged by reminders about the dangers in our body. There it is, overhead, obliterating the sky, that billboard with a carton of cottage cheese, a measuring tape, a scale—this promise of redemption from the disaster of having been made woman. And then, reaching home, still despairing about our size nine jeans, we evoke the most powerful of these voices, because it comes from our own generation, where such a vision would seem impossible. This voice from Susan Griffin's *Woman and Nature:* "On this day we met a woman who was used to getting what she wanted. She ate large portions and her body was big. She let us know there were other such women. We were bewitched. We began to dream we were like this woman."[7]

Now, at last, we are in the house. We are safe here, we suppose, where no one can behold us in our failure to fit into the clothes that have been made too small for us and seem tailor-made to the measure of an adolescent girl. We sit down at the kitchen table, with a cup of coffee and the daily newspaper, hoping to relax from the reawakened horror about the size of ourselves, wondering what it means that in our culture today the entire world of fashion seems to be in retreat from all signs of largeness and maturity in a woman. We open the pages of the Macy's advertisement, dated May 11, 1980. Entitled "Living in the U.S.A.," it is filled with pictures of women and men at play, as they model the clothes and attitudes that best fulfill the fashionable vision of America's summer sportfulness. But the first thing that strikes us as we leaf through this magazine of fantasy and ideal shape is the fact that we cannot find a woman in it. The men are there, with broad shoulders, muscular arms, thick necks, powerful bodies—a reminder that a man may become healthy in pursuit of the ideal form America wishes for him, that perfection for him consists of a diet that makes him strong, exercise that makes him powerful, an attitude toward his body that "builds it up" and makes it massive, while the ideal for a woman is impossible for most of us to achieve if we are to remain women and preserve our health. But now something else strikes us in these pictures. The woman who models the shirt with the plaid collar looks perhaps twelve or thirteen years old. Somehow, we know that she is a woman. And yet, we are not certain how we have this knowledge, for she is dressed, in keeping with her build, very much like a little girl. She wears the cutest visored cap on her head, has tucked up her shoulders so that she looks coy, throws her head to one side so that she seems delicate, stands there dainty and chaste in her white pants, shivering it would seem in an excess of childish giggling. Below her, a two-piece terry shorts set is worn by another capering child, who is also in reality a woman, and who wears a baseball cap and is leaping up in the air, one arm raised, her feet lifted off the ground, as if she were a child jumping up to clap her hands over some treat her father has just brought her. And now everywhere in these pages we see this woman-child wearing clothes suited for a small girl; she is as slender as an unripened adolescent, she wears high socks and sneakers, has skinny legs, undeveloped arms, wears little braids, has no breasts, is coy, delightful, eager to please, a delirious child.

Ah yes, we say, but perhaps this is only our interpretation, inspired by the rancor we feel at the fact that these clothes could not possibly fit us; that we would feel absurd in them, that we don't really want to look coy and cute and shiver with giggles, and jump up and clap our hands, and wear little braids, or have undeveloped chests. Perhaps we exaggerate, and this childishness is not really what our culture is after for its women.

Consider then the case of Christine Olman, one of the leading fashion models of our time. Her picture can be seen in *Voque,* in *Bazaar,* in all the leading fashion magazines; she is photographed by the leading photographers, posing in the traditional seductive postures that sell consumer goods in our culture. Nothing unusual about all this we say? But then we look further. A newspaper article appears and then a television program,[8] both talking about a new wave of young models. Suddenly, we are given a look behind the scenes, before the spotlights and cameras have begun to work. We are shown a room filled with people at work on the model, combing her, clothing her, making her up. But this time the labor of these illusion-makers is expended to its uttermost. For the model they are preparing is modeling clothes intended for mature women and she is twelve years old. This roomful of people is at work to transform a little girl into the illusion of a woman.

But what sort of figure in fact emerges when this labor of transformation has been accomplished? Is it a precociously full-bodied girl who actually looks like a mature woman? Not at all. What emerges is a preadolescent girl, with slender arms and shoulders, undeveloped breasts and hips and thighs, whose body has been covered in sexy clothes, whose face has been painted with a false allure and whose eyes imitate a sexuality she has, by her own confession, never experienced. And this, says fashion, is what a mature woman should attempt to look like.

"It's disgusting," says the photographer who makes his livelihood recording the ideal form of a woman in this land. "It's not necessary," he says, "to have a twelve-year-old look. But that's the look that's selling right now. And Christine is one of the hottest young models around."

It might be redundant to spell out the implicit message in all this, but it can't hurt to state, with all the literalness possible in language, the lesson we are meant to learn as women studying the fashions deemed appropriate for us. According to fashion, large size, maturity, voluptuousness, massiveness, strength, and power are not permitted if we wish to conform to our culture's ideal. Our bodies, which have knowledge of life, must undo this fullness of knowing and make themselves look like the body of a precocious child if we wish to win the approval of our culture.

In Marilyn Monroe we have a transitional figure. A woman permitted to carry large breasts and thighs and hips, to wear tight dresses, to show off her body for the admiration of the entire world, but at the same time required to have an adolescent innocence about her, a pouting coyness, the smile of a little girl.

Laurence Olivier, apparently taken in by Monroe's public persona, believed that she might actually be innocent of sexual knowledge.[9] But Marilyn was a brilliant woman. She knew what her culture wanted of a woman and she knew what to offer when she wished to be noticed or admired. Susan Strasberg tells us that one day when she and Marilyn were walking down the street together, Monroe, who did not always look like her famous self, decided to become "M.M." Suddenly, she was recognized. "Heads turned as they had the first time I had seen her," Strasberg says. "People began to converge on us. She smiled like a little girl."[10]

The smile of the little girl became for Marilyn Monroe the distinguishing characteristic of her public personality, as essential to her fame as her much celebrated body. Most pictures of the actress express this fundamental contradiction that is so essential to our culture—the reassuring vulnerability of a child in the evocative body of the world's most beautiful woman. In Twiggy, and in the anorexic girls modelled upon her, we encounter the further evolution of this tendency already apparent in Monroe. The requirement that women remain arrested in development becomes more visible and more severe. From Mae West to Marilyn to Twiggy to Christine Olman there is a definite progression. If the tendency continues, who knows? We might soon be calling back Margaret O'Brien to model the cultural ideal by which we measure what is required of us as women.

9. WHY NOW?

> A woman should never give the impression that she is so capable, so self-sufficient, that she doesn't need him at all. Men are enchanted by minor, even amusing frailties. This quality of vulnerability, of needing a man, is something that the mature woman should study very carefully. Because it's that quality that she loses most easily. Years of dealing with home and family, of making decisions, of coping, can turn the woman of forty-plus into a brusque, cold-eyed, and somewhat frightening figure. —Gloria Heidi

Is IT A CONSPIRACY, unknown even to those who participate in it?

A whole culture busily spinning out images and warnings intended to keep women from developing their bodies, their appetites, and their powers?

Maybe, when we see another calorie counter on the stand, or read of another miracle diet in a women's magazine, or pick up another container of low-calorie cottage cheese, we must begin to understand these trivial items symbolically and realize that what we are purchasing is the covert advice not to grow too large and too powerful for our culture.

Maybe, indeed, this whole question of the body's reduction is analogous to the binding of women's feet in prerevolutionary China?*

"My mother buys me a girdle when I am fifteen years old," says Louise Bernikow, "because she doesn't like the jiggle. . . . Tighter. I hold myself tighter, as my mother has taught me to do. . . . Is the impulse to cripple a girl peculiar to China between the eleventh and twentieth centuries? The lotus foot was the size of

*Alice Walker, in a conversation about women and their body, suggested this analogy to me.

a doll's and the woman could not walk without support. Her foot was four inches long and two inches wide. A doll. A girl-child. Crippled, indolent, and bound."[1]

There is a relationship between the standards set for women's beauty and the desire to limit their development. In the name of a beautiful foot, the women of China were deprived of autonomy and made incapable of work. A part of the body was forced to remain in a childish condition. They did not walk, they hobbled. In the name of beauty they were crippled.

What happens to women today in the name of beauty?

I'd never wear a girdle, she said,
just medieval throwbacks
to whale baleen brassieres 'n
laced-up waist confiner corsets.
We burned em in the sixties,
girdles, she said walking
into Bloomingdales, grabbing
a pair of cigarette-legged
tight denim jeans off the rack.
Hoisting them up to her hips,
how do ya get em on, she said,
have surgery, take steam baths,
slimnastic classes'n Dr. Nazi's
diet clinic fatshots for a month?
These aren't jeans for going
to lunch in, she said trying
to do the snap, these
aren't even jeans
for eating an hour
before ya put em on, just
for standin up in without
your hands in the pockets,
there's not even room
in here for my underpants.
One hour later she returns
to the store for a new zipper,
front snap, and the side seams
re-stitched. These're jeans

for washing in cold water only
then wearin round the house
til they dry on yr shape,
put em in a clothes dryer,
she said, and you'll get
all pinch bruised
round the crotch'n
your stomach covered
with red streak marks
cross the front.

We burned em in the sixties,
girdles, she said.[2]

We must not imagine that it is only the fashion industry that is upset about the large size of our bodies. Fashion creates and it reflects. Creates, as we have seen, an image few women in this culture are able to realize for themselves. Creates longing—and we all know this longing to win the approval of our culture even at cost to our health, our identity as women, our experience of pleasure in our bodies. But fashion also reflects hidden cultural intentions, as it did in China with the binding of women's feet. As it does in our own day, with pants so tight they serve as an adequate replacement for the girdles that used to bind us. Fashion, for all its appearance of superficiality, is a mirror in which we can read the responses of conventional culture to what is occurring, at the deepest levels of cultural change, among its people.

For instance: if the problem of body and mind is as old in this culture as I have suggested, why is anorexia a new disease and bulmarexia a condition first named during the 1970s? Why for that matter is Christine Olman a model now and not twenty years ago when Marilyn Monroe inspired our admiration?

These questions may help us to understand that something has happened in our culture during the last twenty years that has made us particularly uneasy about the abundance of our flesh. Something, unnamed as yet, which fashion expresses as a shift from the voluptuous to the ascetic.

I wish to place before us a cluster of related facts that constitutes an important cultural synchronicity.

FACT: During the 1960s Marilyn Monroe stood for the ideal in feminine beauty. Now Christine Olman represents that ideal.

FACT: During the 1960s anorexia nervosa began to be a widespread social disease among women.

FACT: During the late 1960s and early 1970s bulmarexia began to be observed as a condition among women.

FACT: During the 1960s Weight Watchers opened their doors. In 1965 Diet Workshop appeared, in 1960s Over-Eaters Anonymous, in 1966 Why Weight, in 1968 Weight Losers Institute, in 1969 Lean Line.

FACT: During the 1960s the Feminist Movement began to emerge, asserting woman's right to authority, development, dignity, liberation and above all, power.

What am I driving at here? I am suggesting that the changing awareness among women of our position in this society has divided itself into two divergent movements, one of which is a movement toward feminine power, the other a retreat from it, supported by the fashion and diet industries, which share a fear of women's power.

In this light it is significant that one of the first feminist activities in our time was an organized protest against the Miss America Contest and the idea of feminine beauty promulgated by the dominant culture through this pageant, in which women strut and display their bodies, as men sit passively, judging them. It is interesting, further, that as a significant portion of the female population in the last two decades began to go to consciousness-raising groups and to question the role and subservience of women in this society, other women hastened to groups where the large size of their bodies was deplored. The same era gave birth to these two contradictory movements among women.

Yet we sense that there is an underlying similarity of motive in both movements. In both, women are driven to gather together and make confessions and find sisterly support for the new resolutions they are taking. In both, women have created new forms of social organization, apart from the established institutions of the dominant culture.

There is, however, also a fundamental divergence here. The groups that arise among feminists are dedicated to the enlargement of women. Confessions made in these groups reveal anger over rape and the shame women have been taught to feel about their bodies; there is interest in the longing to develop the self, concern for the boredom and limitations of motherhood, acknowledgement of the need for sisterly support in the resolution to return to work, go back to school, become more of oneself, grow larger. But in the other groups, confessions are voiced about indulgence in the pleasures of eating, and resolutions are made to control the amount of food consumed, and sisterly support is given for a renewed warfare against the appetite and the body.

Listen to the spontaneous metaphor that finds its way into the discussions of these two groups. In the feminist group it is *largeness* in a woman that is sought, the *power* and *abundance* of the feminine, the assertion of a woman's right to be taken seriously, to *acquire weight,* to *widen* her *frame* of reference, to be *expansive, enlarge* her views, *acquire gravity, fill out,* and *gain* a sense of self-esteem. It is always a question of *widening, enlarging, developing* and *growing.* But in the weight-watching groups the women are trying to *reduce* themselves; and the metaphoric consistency of this is significant: they are trying to make themselves *smaller,* to *narrow* themselves, to become *lightweight,* to lose *gravity,* to be-*little* themselves. Here, emphasis is placed upon *shrinking* and *diminution, confinement* and *contraction,* a *loss* of pounds, a *losing* of flesh, a *falling* of weight, a *lessening.*

These metaphoric consistencies reveal a struggle that goes beyond concern for the body. Thus, in the feminist groups the emphasis is significantly upon liberation—upon release of power, the unfettering of long-suppressed ability, the freeing of one's potential, a woman shaking off restraints and delivering herself from limitations. But in the appetite control groups the emphasis is upon restraint and prohibition, the keeping of watch over appetites and urges, the confining of impulses, the control of the hungers of the self.

When all other personal motives for losing weight are stripped away—the desire to be popular, to be loved, to be successful, to be acceptable, to be in control, to be admired, to admire one's self—what unites the women who seek to reduce their weight is the fact that they look for an answer to their life's problems in the control of their bodies and appetites. A woman who walks through the doors of a weight-watching organization and enters the women's reduction movement has allowed her culture to persuade her that significant relief from her personal and cultural dilemma is to be found in the reduction of her body. Thus, her decision, although she may not be aware of it, enters the domain of the body politic and becomes symbolically a political act.

It is essential to interpret anorexia nervosa, that other significant movement among women during the last decades, so that it, too, can be understood as part of women's struggle for liberation during the last decades. Indeed, Hilde Bruch calls it a new disease because in the last fifteen or twenty years it has occurred at a "rapidly increasing rate." From 1960 on, she writes, "reports on larger patient groups have been published in countries as far apart as Russia and Australia, Sweden and Italy, England and the United States."[3]

The fact that these are highly developed industrial countries, and that anorexia occurs primarily among girls of the upper-middle class, should remind us that anorexia is a symbolic illness. Where hunger is imposed by external circumstances, the act of starvation remains literal, a tragic biological event that does not serve metaphoric or symbolic purposes. It is only in a country where one is able to choose hunger that elective starvation may come to express cultural conflict or even social protest.

"You go over to the high school today and it's like walking into a concentration camp," says the mother of an anorexic girl, in a telephone conversation with a friend, whose daughter has just lost fifty pounds in five months. "Betty Talbot has the same problem, I understand. . . . And of course you know about Kimmy Sanders, don't you? That absolutely gorgeous girl. What a tragedy."[4]

This conversation between mothers, about their anorexic daughters, would not have been heard during the 1950s, or only in rare and isolated cases. Today, however, we may expect to find this conversation in most affluent communities, where families raise daughters who are not able to express their angers and rebellions directly, yet who feel a distinct reluctance to become the conventional people their mothers are.

"Ugh, wretched curves," says the daughter of the mother whose telephone conversation we have just overheard. "I grab my breasts, pinching them until they hurt. If only I could eliminate them, cut them off if need be to become as flat-chested as a child again. It is better now than before I started dieting. To think that I needed a size B bra! Now I don't even need to wear one, but the womanly outline still remains, and I'm afraid that if I should gain again they'll blow up like zeppelins. I would probably start having periods again as well. I would probably look and function just like my mother."[5]

Anorexia nervosa speaks exactly the same protest being spoken by the women's liberation movement. Feminists, it is true, in an outspoken gesture of refusal to comply with the conventional expectations for a woman in this culture, take off their bras. The anorexic girl starves herself instead, so that she does not develop the breasts that would require the bra. The underlying emotional attitude of anorexia is clear: "I don't want to be an imitation," says the anorexic girl. "I don't want to be a victim of fate. . . . I want to make my own name, cut my own image, set my own trend. I want to surpass [my mother], not follow her lead."

This rebellious attitude toward the mother seems to be directed less against the personal mother, more against the limitations of woman's social destiny. Indeed, the mothers of anorexic girls "had often been career women, who felt they had sacrificed their aspirations for the good of the family. In spite of superior intelligence and education, practically all had given up their careers when they married." Their daughters feel impatience with their mothers, dreading that they will share their mothers' fate, which one anorexic girl characterizes in the following way: "to be a nothing, to be devoted to a husband, to be devoted to her children, but without a life of her own."[6]

We might expect that a girl with these attitudes would go out and join a women's consciousness-raising group, discover the alternatives to being what her mother is, and select some form of autonomous, self-fulfilling existence. Unfortunately, however, the typical anorexic girl is, like the heroine of *Edible Woman,* dutiful and submissive; she sees it as a "basic rule of life" to please and not to give offense.[7] Indeed, the private protest we saw earlier in Marian MacAlpin we now see on a widespread, social scale in the anorexic girl. She, too, is a considerate person, who has difficulty forming her own judgments and opinions. Consequently, we cannot expect that she would be able to go to her parents and directly speak her worry and concern about what has happened with her mother's life. Whatever protest she feels must be hidden. And thus her rebellion is expressed through a veiled and disguised symbolism. For it is clear that any other, more positive feminine assertion, beyond the limitations forced upon a growing girl in this culture, are simply not available to her as long as she is determined to please her family. Like Marian, she is doomed to submissiveness, even in her act of protest; her protest itself must be limited to her body—to a refusal and negation of its appetites and its nature. A refusal to eat. A refusal to become a woman.

Anorexic girls continue to get good grades, they graduate with honors from their high schools, but they sit on the stage in all the terrible, mute eloquence of their rebellion. This is how an anorexic girl, looking at her high school graduating class, describes them: "Nan, so frail these days, looks as though she's ready to pass out"; Candy, who has been "released from the hospital on the condition that she gain ten pounds by the end of the month"; Kim, "wraithlike and miserable, her ghostly eyes staring vacantly toward the speaker's podium."[8]

In America of the 1970s and 1980s, no woman can possibly remain unaware of the fact that significant numbers of her sisters are asserting their rights to autonomy, to power, to the development of their full emotional and creative capacities. This movement of women into their enlargement is likely to affect her in a number of ways. She may grow depressed with the life she is living and rebel against it. She may refuse to recognize that her life depresses her and fail to develop a meaningful analysis of her condition as a woman. Or she may feel the force of these contradictory tendencies and enact her entire response to them through her body.

Let us imagine then that a woman comes to awareness of her condition one day in 1969. She is, let us say, forty-five years old, she wears old, dreary clothes, and she is seriously depressed. She is a woman who has tried to diet and failed and who has exhausted her tolerance for weight-watching groups. For her the anorexic solution is simply not a possibility. And so she decides to join a women's consciousness-raising group. There, she tells the other women that her husband has just left her after twenty-five years. She tells how she is stuck in a job with a poverty wage in an insurance company, how she feels a thousand years old. She blames herself, she says, and the fatness in her body, for everything that has gone wrong with her life. But now, because she is encouraged to talk and because no one here believes her rounded belly is the cause of these complex failures, she speaks about a dream she had once as a young girl when she wished to become a writer. She tells how absurd this old dream seems now and how she is afraid. But because the women listen to her fears and encourage her to speak further, she goes home and she begins to dream that she might want to dream of becoming a writer.

Let us also imagine that another similar woman comes to a group intended to help women change their lives. But here, in fact, we do not have to provide the script, for the story of a middle-aged woman named Faye has been written for us by Gloria Heidi, in her unintentionally revealing book:

> She was about forty-five years old when she enrolled in my class —a gray, doughy woman in a dreary maroon, half-size dress—a woman who had obviously come to me as a last resort. "Look, my husband Harry has just walked out after twenty-five years. I'm stuck in a poverty-wage, nowhere job at the insurance company. I feel a thousand years old—and look sixty. But I'm determined to be a new me . . . and I want to start by losing this excess weight. After all, now that I've lost Harry"—her eyes filled with tears— "what else have I got to lose?"[9]

In this group, where the woman comes with a complex social and personal situation, her terrible despair is attributed to the fact that she is fat. She is therefore encouraged to lose weight; a chart is kept of the weight she loses. When the magical transformation finally takes place we are told that the horror of her personal and social position has miraculously altered. A moral is drawn. We are assured that we, too, if only we will lose weight, can be "filled with energy, go aggressively after a better job and with a new figure, a revitalized personality, and an exciting new social life, [like] formerly dowdy and half-sized Faye, [soon] be sitting on top of the world."

The hidden message in this story is profoundly disturbing. Implicitly, we are asked to believe that if every woman lost twenty-five or thirty pounds she would be able to overcome the misogyny in our land; her social problems would be solved, the business world would suddenly fling wide its gates and welcome her into its privileges. Isn't it incredible? We, as women, need only lose weight and all of us will find jobs equal in authority and status and salary to those of men? The need for the Equal Rights

Amendment will vanish? Unemployment figures will dissolve and the very structure of our society will be transformed?

There is a profound untruth here and a subversion of the radical discontent women feel. In a class of this sort, women are directed to turn their dissatisfaction and depression toward their own bodies. They are encouraged to look at their large size as the cause of the failure they sustain in their lives. Consider what it means to persuade a woman who is depressed and sorrowful and disheartened by her entire life, that if only she succeeds in reducing herself, in becoming even less than she already is, she will be acceptable to this culture which cannot tolerate her if she is any larger or more developed than an adolescent girl. The radical protest she might utter, if she correctly understood the source of her despair and depression, has been directed toward herself and away from her culture and society. Now, she will not seek to change her culture so that it might accept her body; instead, she will spend the rest of her life in anguished failure at the effort to change her body so that it will be acceptable to her culture.*

We should not be misled by the fact that we feel more at home in our culture when we lose weight. It may indeed happen that a woman becomes more attractive to men, finds it easier to get a job, experiences less discrimination, receives fewer gibes from strangers, and endures far less humiliation in her own family. Culture rewards those who comply with its standards. But we have to wonder what cost the woman is paying when she sacrifices her body in this way for the approval of her culture. Is she, like the Edible Woman, divorcing herself from her authentic power and identity as a woman? Is she, like Lady Oracle, when she finally loses weight, solving a superficial problem but leaving her essential anguish unresolved? Is she, like most of us, giving up an important source of pleasure? Is she covertly sacrificing other appetites and strivings, other urges and desires associated with the free exercise of her natural self?

*Adapted from a very similar utterance by Louise Wolfe, "The Politics of Body Size," Pacifica Tape Library.

It is only when we cease to trivialize our bodies and our feelings about our bodies that we begin to appreciate how powerful a tool against the development of women is daily exercised by this conventional orientation, which assures us that our sufferings and our depressions are caused by the recalcitrant behavior of our bodies—by their insistence upon feeding themselves, by their unsuppressible urges and wantings and desires, which make us fat.

For what happens when the woman gains back the weight? (Ninety-eight percent of women who have lost weight gain it back.)

What happens when she gains back even more than she lost? (Ninety percent of women gain back more weight than they ever lost.)

What indeed happens to her job and her lover and her new social power and her status in her family and her freedom from the hostility that our culture directs against women who live out their lives in large bodies?

The solution for the woman who eats whenever she feels complex, emotional hungers is exactly the same as the solution for the anorexic girl, who does not wish to become a woman in this culture. Both need to free themselves from the illusion that control of the body's shape and appetites will resolve their dilemma. Both are required to understand that they have reversed problem and solution.

For it happens, again and again, that when the deeper issues are directly engaged, when the anorexic girl makes a connection with her angers and fears, when the fat woman begins to acknowledge the feelings that drive her to eat, the body begins to express this knowledge, takes on the flesh it requires to mature, and gives up those pounds it has been using for the purpose of avoiding feelings. The recognition of this relationship between what we feel and how we look is the only lasting solution to our obsession. Everything else proves to be a transitory and superficial accommodation to the highly suspect, even dangerous aesthetic requirements of our culture. Fat or thin, voluptuous or lean, full or angular, a woman's authentic beauty first comes into existence when her body expresses her self-acceptance—the harmony or the condition of fully conscious creative struggle she has achieved within herself.

Many of us, filled with passionate contradiction at this moment of our emergence, strive indeed to know and develop ourselves as persons and yet simultaneously become obsessed with the control and reduction of our bodies. This paradox, with which we live out our lives, merely underscores the complexity and difficulty of our struggle. It tells us how we may be committed to the idea of our growth and development, while yet in certain, unexamined aspects of ourselves, as we express them through our body, we are still striving for conformity. The behaviors we direct towards the social world may well express our radical orientation towards a woman's self-development. But the behaviors we direct towards our own body express our implicit loyalty to the conventional world.

For we can imagine that a culture based upon the suppression of women will be inclined, precisely in that era when a significant number of women are rediscovering the imagery and meaning of the Amazon, to turn away from whatever is powerful in women. The images in fashion magazines, on billboards, in store windows reflect this turning away from female power, but so also does the masculine retreat from grown women as erotic images. This retreat runs a parallel course to the women's reduction movement and expresses an identical fear of female power. Thus we come upon one final cultural synchronicity. In the era of women's liberation, which is also the era of fat farms and the body's emaciation, popular culture begins to produce movies in which photographers, grown men, become entranced with the Pretty Baby who lives in a whorehouse. In this same era of women's development some two hundred and sixty-four periodicals appear on the marketplace with child pornography.[10] In 1975 Houston police uncover "a warehouse filled with child pornography . . . 15,000 color slides of children, 1,000 magazines, and thousands of reels of film."[11] During this time of the assertion of woman's power we have films like *Taxi Driver,* "in which a twelve-year-old prostitute happily gratifies any male whim in order to please her loathsome pimp. Jodie Foster, who played the adolescent prostitute, was so well received in the role that she soon starred in *The Little Girl Who Lives Down the Lane,* in which she performed as a thirteen-year-old bundle of budding sexuality."[12] In the film *Manhattan* the most popular comedian of his day, a man forty or so, afflicted with an old-fashioned European melancholy and an entirely modern haplessness in the face of existence, turns for comfort and redemption to a seventeen-year-old girl when his wife, a grown woman, leaves him and becomes a lesbian. There is Chester the Molester who seduces little girls and boys as humor in the pages of *Hustler* magazines. And there is the adolescent girl who wrote the following letter to the author of *Kiss Daddy Goodnight,* a book of horror tales of the incest inflicted upon little girls by their fathers. "So if a girl wants my advice now I would say it is OK to do it with Dad until you are about thirteen or fourteen but after that he will lose interest in you and abuse you sexually by letting other people do it up you so it is best to stop at that age, and if I did, then I would still like Dad and not be mad at him like I am."[13]

Naturally, I cannot prove that the masculine preference for little girls is on the increase in our time because grown women are asserting their right to power. The preference itself is not as easy to document as the fact that the women in the fashion magazines are made to look like adolescent children or that the sizes in the clothing stores are growing smaller or that millions of women are attending diet organizations and seeking to reduce themselves while tens of thousands of others cause themselves to vomit every night. I am asking only that we begin to think about these simultaneous events in our cultural life; that we ponder the words of a fifth grade teacher in a city school: "Sexual abuse . . . incest . . . you don't know," she says, "you don't know . . . the kids in my class, the littlest girls . . . the uncles, the brothers, the fathers. It's epidemic and they all cover it up."[14]

Taken together, these words and the books and films and cartoons and letters we have been considering suggest a tendency in which men prefer to encounter little girls instead of grown women. Upon reflection, there is even something highly predictable about this. "Certainly," says Grace Paley, "any culture that prefers women to be childlike and dependent will, with a certain terrible logic, use its children as though they were grown women."[15]

Thus, what we are seeing in this tyranny of slenderness is more than a cultural warfare between body and mind, more even than a bitter struggle against the life cycle and the free expression of our kinship with nature. In this age of feminist assertion men are drawn to women of childish body and mind because there is something less disturbing about the vulnerability and helplessness of a small child—and something truly disturbing about the body and mind of a mature woman.

10. MAN AND WIFE

Where you can, turn to the worst your girl's attractions. . . . Call her fat, if she is full-breasted. . . . —Ovid

It is only the man whose intellect is clouded by his sexual impulses that could give the name of the fair sex to that undersized, narrow-shouldered, broad-hipped, and short-legged race. —Arthur Schopenhauer

Asked whether he believes women have souls, another man answers: "Certainly, if they are not born with them it's a poor creature indeed who can't get one from some man by the time she's eleven years old." —William Faulkner

The fact that the [castration] was self-chosen . . . suggests that men were ready and willing to become "female" in order to share women's superior powers. —Bruno Bettelheim

I OPEN my daily newspaper. I read this letter, signed by a man who calls himself "Depressed" and who reveals indeed all the symptoms of a considerable anguish. He writes:

> Dear Abby:
> I've composed this letter hundreds of times in my mind. I don't know where else to turn. My wife gained ten to 15 pounds while pregnant with our son 11 years ago. She has never been able to lose that weight despite many dieting attempts. Instead she has gradually gained additional weight until now she has a very conspicuous pot belly. In addition, she gets very little exercise, so she tends to doze off about 8 p.m. every evening. I weigh the same as when I graduated from college. I have tried every method I can think of to encourage her to lose weight—incentives, insults, praise, punishments, joint exercise, and threats. We even separated over this a few years ago. Otherwise she is a great wife and wonderful mother. I do love her, and have no desire to see our

> marriage end. However, I cannot accept her as she is no matter how hard I try. Neither can I understand her lack of pride concerning her physical appearance. This problem is continually on my mind, and I am afraid that a permanent separation will eventually be the result. Am I being selfish and unreasonable?
>
> —DEPRESSED

Abby answers this letter in the following way. "Dear Depressed," she writes: "Yes. If you love your wife and are sincere when you say you have no desire to see your marriage end, you will see a therapist to find out why you can't accept her as she is. You could have a problem that is more serious than hers."[1]

I agree. To me, too, it seems that the man who has grown seriously depressed by his wife's weight has a serious problem. I only wish that I myself could have written back to him. I see so many things in this letter I would love to point out to him. The way, for instance, he punishes and threatens his wife—it seems such extreme, even cruel behavior to direct toward a woman who has become pregnant and gained a little weight. I would like to tell him how much sympathy I feel for this woman who, in the face of his terrible pressure, has failed again and again to lose this weight. I might speculate with him about why this has occurred —perhaps, we might agree, it is an assertion of her right to eat, an indifference to her appearance or perhaps even a preference for looking the way she does. After all, I would remind this man, there are people who think that a woman's belly is a thing of beauty, artists who sculpt and painters who paint large women with veneration. But no doubt I would not be able to convince him. He is obsessed by the way his wife looks. Her mature body disturbs him. Although he loves her and is struggling against his repugnance for her he is afraid that he will have to leave her, as he has done in the past. This man has been driven to this extremity by the fact that his wife weighs more than she used to. His obsession with her weight has become the single most determining issue in his marital life.

Evidently, we don't have to look to the fashion magazines or to popular culture to discover that we are being hounded and oppressed so that we will not fall prey to the temptation to like our bodies, in their full maturity, the way they are. The cultural tyranny directed towards our big hips is nearer to home—and unavoidable.

Indeed, it is quite easy to imagine what life must be like for this man's wife. Even when she manages to shut the pages of the magazine, close the cover upon the diet book, ignore the advertisements in the daily newspaper, and avoid the medical profession's concern about her size, there is that daily reminder in her husband's despair that her mature, unmistakably female body is unacceptable. Whatever fascination her body might once have held for her, however mingled with fear and dislike, now it must have become seriously contaminated with his response.

And so she looks at herself in the mirror one day and observes the rounded belly that arouses her husband's disgust. She remembers that when she was a growing girl she was intrigued by this rounding of her belly. It meant that she was becoming a woman. Today, however, it means that her husband may want to leave her.

This transposition of meaning transforms her perception of herself. The sight of her belly now fills her with despair. But she is still eager to please him. She tries on a dress he used to love and notices that it fits a little tighter than it did a few months ago. She is filled with horror, even with fear, as she considers that he will notice this, too, the way the woman in her body is more than ever now revealed. Suddenly she breaks out in a sweat; it has happened before, this sudden rush of heat all over her, although she is not anywhere near to menopause. Her entire body, as she hastily pulls off that dress, is covered with a red blush, making the skin seem to bulge. And it is a flushed, red, anxious face that stares back at her, grimacing. "Oh God," she whispers, her voice rising, becoming shrill, hysterical. "Why didn't I stay on my diet like I promised? Oh God, what will become of me now?"

We go over to talk with this woman, alarmed at her distress.

It is not hard to find her, although no name has been printed in the newspaper. She lives next door to us, across the street and down the block; she works in the same office, rides back on the bus with us from school, lives in our own house and inhabits our own body, making her shame and anguish vocal there.

We speak together; in this particular case she is a neighbor to whom I have lent a book about the experience of being fat in America. When I ask her to give it back to me, she hesitates, tells me she will return it, seems embarrassed, and walks away. A few days later, running into her at the bank, I ask her again for the book, very gently, not wishing to press her if the book has become meaningful and important to her. No, she assures me, she will be delighted to return it. Days pass, the book does not come back to me and finally, one day, she sees me in an empty coffee shop and sits down across from me. She tells me that she cannot find the book. And then, in a rush of words that must have been torment to utter, she explains to me she had hidden it away so that her husband would not see her reading it and associate her with those fat women the book was about.

It wrings the heart; I sit very still, not even breathing now, hoping she will continue to speak with me. "It is the tragedy of our married life," she says finally. And I have heard these words so many times before. "My tragedy," she corrects herself. "I'm sure he doesn't even realize it, but since I gained weight he never takes me out anymore. We've almost stopped entertaining. We lead completely separate lives." Here she makes a nervous gesture with her hand, as if to wipe all this away. "Every day, when he leaves for work, he says to me: 'Stay in the sun and keep to your diet.' "

The woman who whispers this confession to me speaks with a voice that is common in our culture. Thus, another woman, who is not at all fat, says: "Whenever we argue, when the fighting is getting really vicious and mean, he says to me: 'I can't stand your fat ass. If I had to pick one thing to hate about you, believe me, that's it.' " And another woman, who is not fat, says: "I know he's ashamed of me; he used to pick me up at work and come to wait for me outside my office. Now he sits in the car, holding a newspaper over his face, as if he doesn't want anyone to see who it is waiting there for this woman who's become so fat. I ask him about it and he denies it. But then, the minute we start to fight, he sure lets me know." And another woman, who is exceptionally beautiful, says: "Since I gained weight he doesn't want to make love with me." Another woman, "He tells everyone who's meeting me for the first time that I've been under stress and have recently gained weight, that I'm going back on my diet soon. And he always tells them how thin I was when he first met me. If anyone comes to our house he takes out the photograph album and shows them the way I used to look. But I was seventeen years old then, not a mother of three children. I can't look like that all my life." And another woman says: "I'm not kidding. My husband left me because I gained ten pounds. He always had a horror of fat women." And another woman, who is not fat, says: "He always hated his mother. Now he says I look just like her. Since I gained weight he never comes home for dinner anymore. I think he's started to have affairs."

These stories of trouble between husband and wife because of a woman's body are not limited to our contemporary accounts. We can find the same tendency to feel uneasy about a woman's body in the fundamental roots of our culture. A very similar tale was told some thousands and thousands of years ago, at a time when the Hebrew people had not yet shaped the Old Testament from the great number of tales and legends of the oral tradition. This tale, although never included in the official Jewish canon, was popular in its day and speaks with relevance to our own. In it we learn that there was an earlier Eve, who was rejected by Adam because God made the fundamental mistake of allowing Adam to watch "while he built up a woman's anatomy: using bones, tissues, muscles, and glandular secretions, then covering the whole with skin and adding tufts of hair in places." According to the tale, this sight of the making of flesh caused Adam such disgust that even when this woman, The First Eve, stood there in her full beauty, he felt an invincible repugnance. Adam, beholding the creation of Eve as a creature of bone, tissue, muscle, and glandular secretion, could not thereafter accept her as his mate. Thus God, according to the tale, complied with Adam's disgust. He took the First Eve away.[2]

It is possible that Adam's dislike for a woman's body is actually a fear of the natural power that belongs to this body. It is also possible that this same fear informs the dislike our contemporary culture has conceived for mature women.

For consider: This God hid a miracle away in the body of woman—he endowed it with His own creative ability and gave to woman the power to conceive life. From all those bones and tissues and muscles and glandular secretions, he made for the body an awesome knowledge of how to nourish the life to which it had given birth. And therefore, it may be necessary to look for a hidden meaning in this story, for a secret, concealed motive that caused Adam to feel such distress.

The major psychological theory of our culture proposes the idea that women feel a primary envy of the male body—in particular, an envy of the penis. In Freud's account, woman is imagined as anatomically deficient, suffering in her self-esteem because this significant aspect of human anatomy has been withheld from her. We have, as yet, no similarly authoritative analysis of masculine psychology, which posits the fact that men feel a primary envy of the female body—in particular, of the breasts and vagina, which have such an essential relationship to birth and life.

There is, however, evidence that young boys feel a distinct envy for the female body. The analyst Bruno Bettelheim, in his observations of disturbed children at the Sonia Shankman Orthogenic School at the University of Chicago, recorded these statements, made by a seven- and an eight-year-old boy. According to Bettelheim, "each of these boys stated repeatedly, independently of the other and to different persons, that he felt it was 'a cheat' and 'a gyp' that he did not have a vagina. They made remarks such as: 'She thinks she's something special because she has a vagina,' or "Why can't I have a vagina?' "[3]

Such comments were not, however, rare and isolated occurrences. The boys would account for tears in another boy by saying: "I know why he's crying—it's because he wants a vagina." Other boys at the school insisted that they too had vaginas, "refusing to accept the fact that girls have two lower body openings." Other boys of varying ages, who seemed to accept their masculine role, showed nevertheless a distinct "hostility toward female sex characteristics just as violent as those of the boys who wish for vaginas." These boys have "many fantasies about cutting off and tearing out breasts and vaginas." Other boys in the school felt cheated because they could not bear a child.

As it happens, these observations of male envy are not limited to a single school. Bettelheim supports his case with the reports of other scientific observers, who had frequently noticed in boys this same envy of pregnancy. And he speaks finally of boys who felt "tormented by the desire to possess female breasts," and who felt envious of breasts "as sources of power and strength in themselves."

There is, indeed, a riddle repeatedly asked among the boys at this school. "What is the strongest thing in the world?" they wonder. And then they respond: "A brassiere, because it holds two huge mountains and a milk factory."

Girls, apparently, never seem interested in this riddle.

We may wonder, therefore, whether the uneasiness contemporary males feel about large size and maturity in a woman's body exists because the body of a woman has the capacity to call up these primary and violent feelings of envy.

If we refer ourselves to fashion again as a reflection of cultural issues, we may find there a decided tendency to dress women like men. Fashion writers are conscious of this tendency, although they do not examine it for deeper implications. "Often what proves to be newsworthy in women's apparel is related to what's happening in menswear," says the fashion writer Beth Trier. "Knits are No. 1 item, along with the preppy look in men's sportswear and the elegant and tailored Duke of Windsor approach."[4]

There's no doubt that masculine fashions allow women more dignity than those fluffy little-girl clothes which have become so popular in our times. Women tend to find such fashions appealing because male clothes contain the implicit, symbolic promise of conferring upon those who wear them the rights and prerogatives of masculine power. But it is possible that men find them appealing in women because they perform the additional function of stripping away from a woman's body all that might arouse masculine envy.

In the 1920s, when the suffragette movement reached the culmination of its efforts to obtain the vote for women, women were very eager to look like boys. For a woman, the meaning in this shift of fashion is quite different than it might be for a man looking on at this change. A woman, dressing like a boy, binding her breasts, bobbing her hair, is probably asking for freedom, autonomy, and all those rights traditionally reserved for men. Certainly, this right to move freely in masculine society is what male attire meant for George Sand. But this fact should not blind us to the sacrifice involved for a woman here. Masculine culture may occasionally be willing to allow power to a woman if she is willing to sacrifice the qualities that make her distinctively a woman. When we enter masculine culture we are asked to be nonemotional, objective, subdued, more pragmatic in our approach to the world, more instrumental, less involved in the subtleties and nuances of relatedness. We are asked, in short, to model ourselves upon the ideal man in the way we appear and in our behavior.

"I can't walk onto the campus with big breasts and big hips and feel that I belong," says a professor at the University of California. "It's a male institution. I'm voluptuous. And I've always known that voluptuous does not belong at the University."

But what about a woman with big breasts and large thighs,

wearing loose, flowing clothes and bearing the precise mind of a mathematician; a woman scholar who combines the rigorous scientific genius of a biochemist with a poetic passion for subjective truth; a woman who is intensely emotional and has, as a high-placed business executive, that rare capacity to bring a conference room full of disparate individuals together as a group? Women, tucked and abundant, ascetics and celebrants, with hips and asses, breasts and thighs, making deals, weeping, discovering, figuring out, laughing, teaching, inventing, creating, sawing, debating in public, growing angry, hammering nails, with that quality women bring to whatever we do, something of passion, some quality of involvement, an elemental caring for whatever it is in which we are engaged. I am speaking about a woman who is required to sacrifice nothing whatsoever for the privilege of entering culture—a woman who is permitted to carry a developed mind within a fully developed, female body.

Is this possibility regarded as so radical because of the unconfessed masculine envy of women's powers—an envy which boys experience first as a resentment over the fact that in the body of women the mysteries of life and death have been enclosed?

Indeed, we may wonder, further, whether the whole tradition of disparagement of the body arises because of this envy. Maybe Adam, and all the men who followed him, have decided to come to terms with their jealousy about a woman's body by denying the body, as such, any intrinsic worth.

A familiar strategy. Aesop's fox, leaping up for grapes that are beyond his reach and then deciding they must be sour anyway. Adam, watching God close the mystery of life within Eve's body, consumed with envy and driven then to deny value to what he cannot possess. And then, if the desire for the female body, the envy and jealousy, continued to trouble Adam and his descendants, they might take a further step and insist that not only was the body worthless, it actually filled them with disgust.

The little tale we have read becomes a cryptogram, in which Adam's disgust for flesh conceals a profound jealousy, an anger and despair over the miracle of the flesh that was given to woman and withheld from man. And here we must recall that there was once an entire tradition of the ancient Goddess, when the body of a woman inspired veneration and awe. Maybe this story of Adam's early repugnance for the flesh is an attempt to reverse an earlier tradition, in which the body of a woman was the primary sacred object. Maybe the letter writer who is "Depressed" and all the husbands who refuse to take pride in their wives' large size are heirs to this attempt at reversal, which places them at several removes from their authentic response to a woman's body.

But this is true, too, of the women in this culture. In our obsession with our own flesh, in our repeated efforts to strip it of the abundance that arouses male envy, we have unwittingly enrolled ourselves in this troubled tradition of repugnance for the body. And we have allowed the men of our culture to persuade us that this fleshly miracle granted to us through our membership in the female sex is really a cause for shame and despair. Indeed, we have acquiesced in yet a further distortion. For, in our culture, when the attributes are passed out and particular qualities are assigned to particular genders, the body is usually associated with women, and the spirit, the mind, all the "higher" faculties are associated with men.

This apportionment would not be so damaging if the body were regarded as an object of glory, containing wisdoms and wonders equal to or surpassing those of the mind. If we remembered to pay reverence to our own flesh, and to receive instruction from it, as Evelyn Scott does in this beautiful passage, we would indeed have begun to recover an important source of wisdom:

> With my pregnant body it is different. My mind is filled with a kind of stillness of understanding. . . . I believe in myself, just as I believe in things outside me through the objectivity of touch. . . . When I am convinced of something I am convinced under my whole self, *as though my flesh had informed me.* Now I KNOW. Knowledge is the condition of my BEING.[5]

But in a place where our bodies seem to fill everyone with dislike, where their knowledge and wisdom are denied, women must bitterly regret the fact that we are bearing an entire culture's negative burden of fleshly existence. For the fact remains that Adam and "Depressed," although they do not confront this issue directly, are also creatures of bone and tissue and muscle and glandular secretion. And here we must become aware that the male denial of fleshly existence has a long tradition. We must understand that this psychological maneuver, by which an object inspiring jealousy is converted into an object arousing disgust, has even further twistings and turnings within the psyche. For when the body has come to be considered a vile and repugnant thing, it is inevitable that men will wish to deny the fact that they possess a body at all.

There was, for instance, a rabbi in the Middle Ages who asked: "Why must a woman use perfume, when a man does not need it?" And then he answered: "Dust of the ground remains the same no matter how long it is kept, while flesh putrifies without salting."[6]

In our more enlightened psychological times we can recognize the irrationality in this insistence that only the body of a woman putrifies while the dust-originated body of a man merely returns to its original condition. But the irrationality has been forced upon the rabbi, and all those who reason like him, by the fact that no man would wish to possess a body that masculine tradition has come to regard with disgust.

Indeed, how fortunate it would be for a man if it were true that only woman had a corruptible body; through this distinction he could escape all experience of illness and age, the growing feebleness of the body that affects the mind, threatens the continued existence of the soul, and afflicts the spiritual self with the stench of corruption. How comforting it would be for a man if this happened only to his wife, and if our common knowledge of this common fate could be successfully covered over with perfume.

Unfortunately, for women and men both, the situation is not so simple. We all, members of both sexes, have been consigned by our membership in the human race to live out our lives within a body, with all the glories and limitations this imposes upon us.

But men have managed to locate in the body of a woman all the difficulties of life within the body. Apparently, whatever the original childhood experience of the body for both women and men, the men of our time have managed to distance themselves from a direct knowledge, in their own flesh, of all the disadvantages of fleshly existence. And women, for reasons we must investigate further, have accepted this burden of the scapegoat.

Indeed, for the man in this culture, abundance of flesh does not invariably signify that there is something wrong with him and that he has become, for those who love and cherish him, a source of shame. Even when he gains a great deal of weight, becomes what we regard as fat and therefore asserts the undeniable fact of fleshly existence, we do not shrink away from him and find him an object worthy of scorn. There is, for instance, the fat man, most familiar in this culture as the millionaire, whose vest bulges and whose gold watch pokes out from his straining pocket, a figure of prestige and influence, whose size reflects his power. "Probably this country will never see again so many fat, rich men as were prevalent at the end of the last century, copper kings and railroad millionaires and suchlike literally stuffing themselves to death in imitation of Diamond Jim, whose abnormally large stomach coincided so miraculously with the period."[7] One cannot imagine a woman taking on this added girth in order to assume with it the associated qualities of power and influence, self-assertion, even the aggrandizement of self, which seemed to accompany the bloated belly of the millionaire. If a woman should grow fat in this way we would see in this augmentation of herself a cause for shame and derision. "Fat women," Marcia Millman writes, arouse in us "horror, contempt, morbid fascination, shame and moral outrage." They experience, as a result of this, extreme forms of social sanctions against their size, suffering from "job discrimination, social exclusion, personal shame and low self-esteem, exploitation by commercial interests, inability to buy most health and life insurance, unsympathetic treatment by doctors, and public ridicule."[8]

Even today, when the sight of a fat man no longer reminds us invariably of Diamond Jim and the railroad millionaires gorging themselves at the turn of the century, it is unlikely that a large man would create the following scene, which I witnessed several weeks ago.

I was wheeling my basket down the aisle of the neighborhood grocery store when I saw a fat woman moving in front of the shelves at the back of the store. She was gathering in food, taking cans from the shelf, filling up her basket. She behaved no differently than anyone else, but it was clear that she had become an object of fascinated interest. There was that highly charged atmosphere in the place, a sense that too much energy had gathered and now would have to be discharged. As she passed, people caught one another's eye, knowing looks were exchanged, a teen-aged boy made an exaggerated show of pressing himself back against the shelves so that he could give her room to pass and a woman standing next to me said: "It's like watching a death's head. The Co-Op ought to pay her to get out of here. Who can go home to a good dinner with that in mind?" At this point the fat woman, walking slowly behind her basket, passed quite close to us, her eyes averted, blushing furiously. "Oh, God, you don't think she heard me?" the other woman whispered to me. "I always think of them as if they're sealed off behind that wall of fat."

I don't know whether the woman overheard this conversation. I am inclined to think she did not, that her averted eyes and flushed cheeks arose from the general atmosphere created by her appearance in the food store. I have seen the same thing in the ice cream parlor, where a fat woman had trouble getting into the booth; and I know that the same laughter and knowing glances will invariably surround the entrance of a fat woman in a revolving door or through a turnstile. And there was the time a child, running down the street, collided with the large belly of a woman walking toward him. People watching this, as they went to pick up the child and to help the woman, whose packages had fallen, covered their laughter as they walked toward her, shoulders shaking. It may be that I feel so much sympathy for these women because I have always imagined that I looked like them; I have walked out on the street, or on the beach, or on the dance floor, feeling that people were casting just such knowing looks at me. But I don't think even I could exaggerate the pain these women suffer because they are large. In the face of their obesity our normal standards of humanity vanish and we are possessed by a form of racist revulsion for the bodies of these women. "I can't stand fat women," a woman says. "If one of them has been sitting on a chair in a coffee shop, or on the bus, and there's no other place to sit, I won't go in there or sit in that place."

By now it must be evident that the fat man has been spared this burden of negative symbolic meaning only because the fat woman has taken it on. One of the great advantages to men, in a culture they dominate, is the ability to assign to those they oppress whatever it is they wish to disown or ignore in their own condition. It is because the fat man believes the imagery his own culture has created that he can gorge himself with impunity and strut about the pool with his bulging belly, while the fat women are all wearing blouses in the water. Because his wife has agreed to carry the general shame our entire culture feels about the body, he can proudly walk up to the younger women who are absorbed in one another's company; and now he insists upon opening conversation with them, his belly neatly held between his proud hands, as if it too were an estimable possession. But his wife feels shame at herself and so, as she gets out of the pool, she instantly covers herself with the robe that has been carefully spread out there, ready to receive her.

When *Hustler* magazine publishes a cartoon, meant to provide us with entertainment, showing a fat person standing on a scale, the person drawn in its pages is a woman with huge breasts and a bulging stomach and a huge ass and swollen calves, with pearls around her fat wrists and carrying a tiny handbag. And we, who can read this cryptograph with initiated eyes, see here, not just the ludicrous portrait of a fat person, but the enormously exaggerated fatness of a woman, which is meant to help us believe that the problems of the flesh are a woman's problem—that this weight and girth and abundance, which make the fact of the body undeniable, are all really appurtenances of the female.

For there is a certain telling note of insistence in all this; it sounds in the diet books and in the warnings of the medical profession and in the church sermons and in the pornographic magazine, and it is repeated in the husband's insistence to his wife, and it was there when Adam was speaking to God. It begins, indeed, to seem that men must remind themselves over and over again that it is women who are the problem here, with their propensity toward fleshly existence and their large bodies that make this propensity evident. But this insistence should remind us that these projections and denials, these relocations of conflict about oneself, are difficult to sustain; they are in danger constantly of collapsing back upon us and exposing the fact that men and women both move about through the world in the "adipose prison" of a body.

Indeed, this whole screen of negative and repugnant imagery of the body is in danger of collapsing altogether and exposing the fact that women carry a body that bears a glory even more than a repugnance. For the female body, which can stand for the undeniable fact of our mortality, can also remind us that only one-half of the human race carries the divine capacity to conceive, to nurture, and to give birth to life.

If we, as a culture, were able to tolerate this fact, we might also be willing to let women grow large, become mature, and carry in pride the natural wonder of the human body in all its abundance.

11. CLUES

> Fantasies of the father, or of himself, ripping up the mother, beating her, scratching her, cutting her into pieces, are some instances of childish conception of intercourse.
>
> —Melanie Klein

> You belong to a type that's very common in this country, Mrs. Phelps—a type of self-centered, self-pitying, son-devouring tigress . . . talk about cannibals!
>
> —Sidney Howard

IDEALS ARE TRICKY and problematic creatures; they keep themselves apart from most of the things we grow curious about and call into question. Often, those cherished most ardently by an age rarely come into the open, where we could direct toward them the critical scrutiny of our changing consciousness. They remain hidden, so close to us that we cannot perceive them. Nietzsche had much to say about this. "Would anyone care to learn something about the way in which ideals are manufactured?" he once asked. "Does anyone have the nerve? . . . Well then, go ahead! There's a chink through which you can peek into this murky shop. But wait just a moment, Mr. Foolhardy; your eyes must grow accustomed to the fickle light. . . . All right, tell me what's going on in there, audacious fellow; now I am the one who is listening."[1]

It is with these words that Nietzsche invited an entire culture to look beneath the surface of its moral judgments, its categories of good and evil, its notions of right and wrong. He was, of course, correct in suggesting the audacity it would require to peek in this way beneath the surface into that murky shop of our hidden motivations. For we, too, in this matter of aesthetic judgment, in our notions that slenderness in a woman is preferable to fat, require eyes accustomed to the fickle light and ears adjusted to the sound of whispering when we approach those depths of the psyche where one thing is transmuted into another.

Consequently, I would like to structure our investigation from this point as if it were part detective story, part the wisdom journey of Goethe's Faust. If we have satisfied ourselves that our culture plays a significant role in encouraging women to disparage their bodies, we must nevertheless still understand the tendency shown by women to accept the negative image our culture assigns to us. For we, who are forever on a diet, seem to be collaborating in these hostile attitudes towards the body, we who have so much reason to glory in the flesh. Otherwise why don't we simply claim, along with all the other rights and powers, the right to our body as nature has endowed it? We are faced with a mystery and our investigation must continue. And so we follow the path of Faust and Mephistopheles as they descend into the mysterious depths where the issues of culture and individual psyche converge. Into the realm of the Mothers we follow them, where Faust encounters a primeval dread:

FAUST: Speak, nor delay thy history!
MEPHISTOPHELES:
Reluctant, I reveal a higher mystery.
In solitude enthroned are goddesses,
No place about them, and of Time still less,
And but to speak of them embarrasses.
They are the Mothers!
FAUST: Mothers!
MEPHISTOPHELES: Hast thou dread?[2]

THE FIRST CLUE:

"Then he found himself. Without his being aware, the street had begun to slope and before he knew it he was in Freedman Town, surrounded by the summer smell and the summer voices of invisible negroes. They seemed to enclose him like bodiless voices murmuring, talking, laughing, in a language not his. As from the bottom of a thick black pit, he saw himself enclosed by cabinshapes, vague, kerosenelit, so that the street lamps themselves seemed to be further spaced. . . .

"He was standing still now, breathing quite hard, glaring this way and that. About him the cabins were shaped blackly out of blackness by the faint, sultry glow of kerosene lamps. On all sides, *even within him,* the bodiless fecundmellow voices of negro women murmured. It was as though he had returned to the lightless hot wet primogenitive Female. He began to run, flaring, his teeth glaring, his inbreath cold on his dry teeth and lips, toward the next street lamp."[3]

This scene, from William Faulkner's *Light in August,* takes us into the nether regions of the psyche. It is set in a Southern town, but it has about it all the atmosphere of a descent into psychological depths and is symbolically equivalent to Faust's journey with Mephistopheles. The man walks toward the pit, where a language other than his own is spoken, the actual presences are not visible, and he hears a murmur of disembodied voices. He is descending into the unconscious, or into Hades, which served the ancient world for the same symbolic journey. What he encounters here, in the sultry glow of kerosene lamps, is terrifying. For it is the original Female, hot, wet, murmuring, and distilled down to a very essence of sensuality.

SECOND CLUE:

Some years ago, I myself dreamt Faulkner's scene. I, too, in my dream, was wandering in an unfamiliar part of town and came to a place lit by a gaslamp, where the houses were old and the dwellings existed beneath the level of the street. From one of these I heard music, the sound of laughing voices, I could smell perfume and was aware of a scent of musk, or sex, or the unimaginable permission for sensual pleasure. I went toward the place, knocked at the door. A huge woman answered it; she was naked and her dark skin seemed to glisten in the light of the lamp from the street. I wanted to run away, but she took my hand and drew me inside. There were only women in this place, dancing together, eating and drinking, laughing, combing each other's hair, putting oil on their bodies, lying together, writhing and groaning. They were all large women, much larger than life-size. I felt an incredible longing to be with them, to lie with them. But my terror was overwhelming. I broke out in a sweat, I pulled away from the woman. She drew me back, pressed my head to her breasts, as if I were an infant and she were offering me suck. I felt she was trying to smother me. Somehow, I got away from her, I raced outside but then, unaccountably, even as I was running, I stopped to look back. I wanted to remember the name of the street so that I could get back to the place. I stared and stared at the street sign, still gasping for breath, but I knew already that the way was lost. I would awaken, I would be unable to make my way back to that unfamiliar part of town.

Because I am a woman, my terror in this dream was cut through with longing and regret. But there can be no doubt that what filled me with so much fear was this vision of the Female. For I am suggesting that we, the women of this culture, share the fear of women and natural existence that inspires our culture generally.

In *Pornography and Silence,* Susan Griffin has shown that our culture, and the psyche which produces it, tend consistently to associate both women and Blacks with the body, with instinct and with sensuality, and to fear both women and Black people because of this association.[4] The fear of nature is thus an influential fear, inspiring the horror of racism and the repression of women. For we hunt down, suppress or attempt to inflict harm upon whatever might call us back to nature, whether this call arises from our own body or from a people to whom we have attributed those qualities of instinctual life we wish to separate from ourselves. In this sense it is possible to see a psychological similarity between the tyranny of slenderness and the fear of women; just as there is a common ground between the will to starve the flesh and the racist attitude. However diverse these phenomena at first sight appear, they are together influenced by a fear of natural existence.

It is thus no accident that Faulkner's story makes a symbolic association between being Female and being Black. No accident either that the same association is apparent in my dream. A woman who dreads what is natural and sensual in herself assigns these urges to her body and then tries to starve and purge them out of existence. When she begins dreaming, and encounters her own desire again, her psyche will employ the imagery generally available in her culture.

But our work here is very difficult. The audacity Nietzsche spoke of is more than ever required now. For there broods over this topic of our culture's fear of women what Wolfgang Lederer has called a "strange silence." In his research into the psychoanalytic studies on the fear of women, Lederer found very little available material. He went to the *Index of Psychoanalytic Writings* from 1965 back to the "beginnings of Psychoanalytic time"; he researched the *Psychological Abstracts,* back to 1927; and he examined, of course, the *Collected Works of Freud.* He reports his findings in this way:

THIRD CLUE:

> . . . under the index headings: "Women, fear of"; or: "Women, men's fear of" we encounter amazingly little. *The Psychoanalytic Index* shows three listings—one an article in a popular magazine, one little more than a brief clinical note dated 1932. The abstracts contain two items: an Adlerian paper by Branchfield dated 1928, and another, also listed in the Index, by Karen Horney. In this paper, entitled "The Dread of Woman" and dated 1932, Horney, having examined ample clinical, mythological and anthropological evidence, exclaims: "Is it not remarkable that so little recognition and attention are paid to the fact of man's secret dread of women?" And her amazement, justified in 1932, would be as valid today. No flood of amplification has followed her remarks, no band of clinicians has staked a claim on what would seem to be a clinical Klondike . . . the topic of the fear of women is today, in psychoanalytic writings, as neglected as ever. . . .[5]

Lederer wrote this in 1968; since then feminist thinkers have begun to record evidence of this fear of woman. But little has changed in the *Psychoanalytic Index.* There, where tradition holds sway, little has been added to break this strange silence Lederer observed.

Consequently, I should not be surprised to discover this same silence in myself. How many times I have turned away from this work feeling calmly persuaded that I had glimpsed an important, hidden truth, only to feel, an hour or two later, that I was walking the edges of absurdity. I have found that, in the face of this resistance, no insistence or rhetorical flourish can avail. What I needed, and what I must here provide, is a gathering of suggestive evidence, a turning of thought in a particular direction, where insights, formerly withheld from awareness, can become available: Faulkner's vision of this descent into the primordial Female; my own dream, which I remember when I read Faulkner's work; and now this collection of mythic associations to the destructive power of woman.

FOURTH CLUE:

> The Sphynx, with her riddles, was a throttler of men. Echidna, half a young woman with bright eyes and fair cheeks, half a snake dwelling in the depths of the earth and eating raw meat, killed all men who happened to come her way. . . . Her daughter Scylla, once a beautiful woman but changed into a monster with six fearful heads and twelve feet, sitting in a cave opposite Mount Aetna, seized all the sailors who passed through the straits of Messina, cracked their bones and slowly swallowed them; she did this, of course, provided that they did not first get sucked in by that other voracious woman, the whirlpool Charybdis, the "sucker down," a daughter of Mother Earth. . . .[6]

There is something about this imagery that awakens a responsive chord; something has been recorded here which begins to explain our fear of woman. For this fear seems driven to elaborate itself, over and over again, in terms of the same imagery. These fearful she-monsters not only destroy men: they eat, they swallow, they suck. They are voracious. This image of woman as destructive seems inextricably involved with the idea of eating. And this thought in turn suddenly reminds me: it was through our own, infantile hunger that woman was first known to us. It was we ourselves who, in our first encounter with the female, ate and swallowed and sucked. We ourselves were the voracious ones. It was we who were once the primordial hunger we have since attributed to woman.

And so perhaps it is possible to expand this idea, to enlarge it as a general notion, that in our relations to women we have a tendency to attribute to them what we ourselves once felt toward them, making them responsible for all our hungers, for any destructive wishes we might have conceived toward them during our infancy, attributing to them all of our insatiable desires, as in this story, which was told to the anthropologist Malinowski by a Trobriand native.

FIFTH CLUE:

> Far away, beyond the open sea . . . you would come to a large island. . . . There are many villages. Only women live in them. They are all beautiful. They go about naked. They don't shave their pubic hair. . . . These women are very bad, very fierce. This is because of their *insatiable desire.* When sailors are stranded on the beach, the women see the canoes from afar. They stand on the beach awaiting them. The beach is dark with their bodies, they stand so thick. The men arrive, the women run towards them. They throw themselves upon them at once. The pubic leaf is torn off; the women do violence to the men. . . . They never leave the men alone. There are many women there. When one has finished, another comes along. When they cannot have intercourse, they use the man's nose, his ears, his fingers, his toes—the man dies.[7]

From the Trobriand native to Faulkner's hero in *Light in August* to the dream of a contemporary woman is quite an arc, and it spans, in fact, an extraordinary amount of psychological history. For this violent, insatiable desire the Trobriand imagined in his island of women finally carries us back to the primordial moment our clues have been reaching for.

Finally, we have arrived at those "deepest depths" where Faust was led by Mephistopheles. We too have come to the realm of the Mothers and like Faust, confronting the Rape of Helen, we must now be willing to behold an image of our secret desire (held in common with our entire culture) to take possession of a woman's body by force. For this idea of taking possession can be elaborated at an even deeper psychic level, through the imagery of violent, insatiable desire. And we, who know something about insatiable desire, must ask ourselves now what the body of a woman must have looked like to a small infant—the huge breasts, the belly rounded and swelling, the thighs so large and abundant. Once, at the very beginnings of existence, there was a time when all insatiable desire was turned upon this body of a woman and this body must have seemed then a veritable mountain of flesh.

Clearly, this one fact alone must have a great deal to do with the reasons we are so resistant to large size in a woman; and this almost forgotten fact from our earliest childhood must have something to do with our tendency to blame women for what goes wrong in our life, and for our mortality, and to assign to woman our own struggles over our bodies and appetites. For once, this huge, Female presence, called the mother, was responsible for the frustration of our limitless, our violent, our insatiable desire.

It is no wonder that Mephistopheles is reluctant to speak of the Mothers. No wonder that the descent of Faulkner's hero into the hot wet ooze of the primogenitive Female awakens so much dread in him. Even the imagery narrating this descent seems to reach back to the physical experience of the first moments of existence, when we arrived and stared out at the world, wailing between a woman's oozing legs. It is no wonder, either, that my own dream repeats this same dread and terror of the first knowledge of the feminine. Every woman in this culture shares with every man the same primordial experience of woman. For both, woman was once all in all the world to us.

But why hadn't we seen that before? What we first knew of life and existence we first knew as woman's body. How extraordinary this seems. Everything we first felt and touched and tasted and ate—all sensual knowledge—was of a woman's body. No wonder sensuality still means woman to us; no wonder the "bodiless voices murmuring" rise up to us from the Mothers' realm. The first voice in our ears was the voice of woman whispering; the first knowledge in our hands, of skin and hair, of the shape of round and curved, was sensual knowledge of woman. And the smell of milk, the taste of skin, the way anger and hunger smells was woman.

If we have, unexamined or unconfessed, a problem with woman that makes us prefer her reduced in size and of lesser gravity, this must have something to do with the awesome girth and power of a woman during the first moments and years of our existence. However small the mother was in fact, to her infant, cast adrift and turning to this body for its home, she must have seemed gigantic.

12. THE PRIMORDIAL FEMALE

> We find that the child feels, when the breast is wanted but is not there, as if it were lost forever. —Melanie Klein

> I cried out. "See what you have done, you wretches, you robbers, you ghouls feeding on breasts; see, see what you have done."
>
> —Renée, *Autobiography of a Schizophrenic Girl*

> Is it the great beauty she hears a lullabye/a wide song a lap. . . . —Francis Jaffer

THIS INSIGHT opens upon a lost world. And it explains also the anxiety we feel making our way back to this fundamental experience, where world and nature and self and a woman's body all converge in a simultaneous event of birth and awakening. For here we come upon that same infantile experience we have peeked into before, in examining the origins of hatred for our bodies. But now the focus has shifted, and the body we are so passionately involved with here is not our own, but woman's body, the body of the mother, toward which we are turning for survival. We have returned here to an even earlier time than that in which we lay entranced with the movements of our own fingers and toes; and this time must have left a profound mark upon our emotional and psychological life, influencing what we sculpt and paint, influencing also the relations between women and men, between a wife's body and the husband's response to it, and a woman's response to her own body. No wonder then that the issue of our bodies—as they appear to others, as we respond to them ourselves—is so charged and significant. No wonder so much energy has been expended, so many statues carved, so many pages of literature written, so much religious thought and so many books on dieting published, and so many sermons delivered and scales sold because of woman's body. Our preoccupation with it derives from the first moments and hours and years of life. And we understand also how our troubles over the body are even older than our first struggle to control it, and how this first grief about the body must have been learned in a woman's arms and at our mother's breast.

It is essential that we recover this lost world if we are to understand the heartland of our obsession with the female body. Everything we have been examining winds its way back to this fundamental point; it is the center at which the spiral of our investigation finally comes to rest. If we are unable actively to recall what we once experienced at our mother's breast, we must resign ourselves to an imaginative reconstruction of it, wondering what it must have been like to awaken to life through a woman's body. We know that these efforts cannot yield more than a plausible understanding, even though recent psychological thinking has opened this period of childhood, criticizing Freud's theories on infantile narcissism and extending his insights. Mahler, Dinnerstein, Chaderow, and Balint[1] have pioneered the re-examination of infancy. But their theories of "primary love" and "anaclitic love" and "primary object clinging," the careful and painstaking examination of object relations, narcissism and symbiosis, are abstractions from an earliest, highly charged emotional experience, which we must enter again in our imaginations if we are to grasp its relevance to our suffering.

We step down into this murkiest realm—the first moments and hours of life, imagining that the infant, swimming in and out of a womb-state of preconscious existence, wakens to sensation, bursts of light, the feel of the mother's breast against mouth and cheek, the touch of water upon the skin, to something touching the head, the back, to the sense of being contained in the motherbody of the world. All this as we imagine it is a sea of mixed sensation, sight not clearly distinguished from touch or feel or taste, inner and outer not separated from one another, who she was and we were not yet distinguished, the breast our hand closed around not different than the hand closing, the belly on which the cheek lay part of the cheek. If life seemed abundant then, teeming and luxurious, in the arms and upon the breast of woman, as if it were a tropical paradise, where food came magically whenever we needed, it is no wonder that all subsequent sense of richness and fecundity in life seems feminine, so that Tahiti for the painter, when it is meant to represent natural abundance and a return to a freer, more sensual existence, must be painted with the nude bodies of women. It is as if this earliest time were continually calling us back to it, lifelong, through the evocative power of whatever is associated with woman.

And now we can imagine the periods of consciousness growing, the sensations threading themselves together, becoming fixed and permanent impressions, so that the hand we look upon remains a hand and does not dissolve again into the light that surrounds it, or become a head moving toward us, or a breast toward which we are ourselves moving. But even these more permanent impressions are influenced by our perception of a woman's body, from which neither the self nor the world have been yet clearly distinguished, so that, older now and looking up, we think she has drawn a blue sky behind her head or a tree to look over her shoulder—she, who is limitless in her power.

It is a time of life in which woman is the universe, her body our source of life and comfort, our paradisical playground of delight, our feeding and touching and feeling and first seeing and sensing, our reaching out and finding, our knowing, all spun round the softness and fullness and abundance and roundness and hugeness of a woman's body. However small the mother was in fact, to her infant, she must have been the entire world. And so we can imagine that these qualities—of softness and roundness, of gentle touching upon our skin, a sudden burst of light, or largeness in a woman's body—will remind us always of this first time.

We can imagine also a later stage of this ease and comfort with existence, which would not have aroused in us fear of the power of woman to remind us of this time; the child is more fully awake now, and the mother's body can be clearly perceived and becomes then an object of passionate interest. The way it moves and bends, bringing us next to it, placing us upon it, settling us inches away and becoming then visible, as if in close-up—a shoulder, a neck, the arc of the belly—and all this, about which we speculate, suddenly made clear and graphic and known to us through a work of art, when the artist, singularly gifted with the ability to recapture the child's vision, shows us the way the body of woman must have looked to the young child. I speak here of the work of Alfred Stieglitz, when he photographed the naked body of Georgia O'Keeffe.[2] Turning the pages of this book, we come to understand the first rapture of the child's relationship to the mother's body; so many of these portraits seem to have been shot by a camera placed exactly in the position of a small child, lying next to his mother on the bed. There she is, her white garment open at the breast, as if she had just been feeding the infant, her sleeves falling back from her arms, as she raises now her hands to her forehead and looks inward, into that immense distance of her subjectivity. There is a stillness about these portraits, a sense of quiet and poise, of timelessness, as life must have seemed to that child, learning to know woman's body and lying there, lost in wonder of this round flesh. And here she is, in close-up—that photographic equivalent of the original vision of childhood, when the child's face was so close to the body it loved, so that the child saw things magnified, isolated, the head lifted, covered in shadow, the neck with the white gown falling back from it, the tendons bulging, that curtain of hair behind which an entire world disappeared.

And now the artist, pursuing this recovery of the lost childhood vision, offers us page after page of portraits of a woman's hand, and so we understand how these hands must have entranced him as an infant—bringing warmth to him, covering him, reaching out to lift him, touching him, drawing him close, changing him, hovering over him.

These strange, all-powerful beings, the hands of the mother—how they are knotted in their power and so large the infant's entire body can be grasped and held by them. These hands, larger even than the entire circumference of the baby's head, are moving there now in a world of their own, attached to no body, the light falling on them, making them luminous and defining their movement as pattern. And they are reaching up now, touching the breast and then sewing with the same grace and power and competence with which they command and shape and order the entire world.

The great vision of this artist, studying the woman with whom he is in love, captures again the child's first sense of these hands performing their miracles—reaching for things so high they cannot be seen until the hands touch and invent them and bring them down; or those hands straining in some terrible anguish of accomplishment, on which our entire well-being depends; and now, clasped together, as for rest from this primordial labor, they are drawing the white robe over the breasts.

Here is genuinely erotic art, which can afford to behold woman in all her subjectivity and power, for it can endure the return to that original relationship to woman, which we are imagining. How the child lies there, unthinking, utterly receptive, while these impressions embed themselves in the very structure of his mind; their evocative power is never again forgotten, they will endure forever. The way the mother stood up from the bed, this body of hers rising there now like a tremendous pillar, a vast colossus as it looms over us, awesome, immense, filling us with a desire to reach out, to touch it, to take it back to us, to run our hands over its curved surface, to grasp those breasts. And the knowledge of these lines and curves passing into us, so that concavity means always woman, and the pendulous fall means always breast, and large size, girth, immensity in a woman means always mother; and then those more sudden, furtive snatches of sight, the gown falling back, the legs parting, that dark forest of hair, the lips of the vulva parting, every wrinkle and crease of flesh observed in their beauty, and then the legs closing, the arms coming forward, enclosing the breasts we are watching now as they gather fullness and move toward us.

Erich Neumann writes:

> Because the identity of the female personality with the encompassing body-vessel in which the child is sheltered belongs to the foundation of feminine existence, woman is not only the vessel that like every body contains something within itself, but, both for herself and the male, is the "life-vessel as such" in which life forms, and which bears all living things and discharges them out of itself and into the world.
>
> The basic symbolic equation woman-body-vessel corresponds to what is perhaps mankind's—man's as well as woman's—most elementary experience of the Feminine.[3]

These words remind us of the child's coming to know the mystery and power in a woman's body. For no culture has invented, no technology ever approached, the fundamental attainments that are natural to the body with its knowledge of how to bring forth food from itself, to bleed and to heal itself from its bleeding, to conceive and carry life within itself, to bring forth life from itself. Even today the memory of the acquiring of knowledge of each one of these things lives with us still. The bloody cloth in the bathroom, the pregnant woman in the park, the babies fed at the breast on park benches in the spring. The story our mother told us of how we were born, roped to her by an umbilical cord. And we wanted to run away and we wanted to hide from the knowledge that was so much older than her telling and which even in childhood could evoke that earlier time, with its dreamy awakenings, and terrified sleepings, the first knowledge of cold and waking alone in the darkness and hunger and the screaming out for succor in the night. And the coming then of the body with its warmth and comfortings, filling our hands, filling our mouth, filling our eyes. . . .

Woman's body, our first home. Our first knowledge of unfathomable mysteries. The first cause of our innocent suffering when it cast us out of itself.

But what a witch's brew of feeling is here, the ground of an original ambivalence, awe at her power, terror at our own helplessness, a body that comforts us and bleeds, withholds itself, becomes lavishly present again, abandons us daily to the universal void and daily welcomes us again into its warm and rounded softness. In the timeless being of infancy, for eons and eons of the slow growth of separateness and the ego's knowledge of itself, this drama of the loss and return of woman's body fills the entire stage of life. Its absence means terror, its return life.

And so we imagine the child waking and crying out and not being answered, through the eternities of timelessness in which she is living still; and we understand the terror of this moment of knowing, when it is borne in upon us that the mother's body is other than the warm bed and the tucked blanket and the slats of the crib; and is different also than the image of the body, the memory and fantasy of the body; and that this body, external to us, and other, is now beyond reach.

Dorothy Dinnerstein has written cogently of this first experience of woman.

> One basis for our species' fundamental ambivalence towards its female members lies in the fact that the early mother, monolithic representative of nature, is a source, like nature, of ultimate distress as well as ultimate joy. Like nature, she is both nourishing and disappointing, both alluring and threatening, both comforting and unreliable.
>
> She is the source of food, warmth, comfort, and entertainment; but the baby, no matter how well it is cared for, suffers some hunger or cold, some bellyaches or alarming sudden movements or unpleasant bursts of noise, some loneliness or boredom, and how is it to know that she is not the source of these things, too?[4]

In this primordial drama we have discovered a reason not to remember the broken paradise of first knowledge of a woman's body. For this is a time filled, not only with warmth and softness and comfortings, but with memories of terror and waking in anguish, and the learning of our own powerlessness to command the world, and the learning too of our own helplessness, our dependency upon the body of woman.

So much has vanished in this moment of terror—our earliest sense of power and oneness with the world, an earlier stage of omnipotence, when our fantasies seemed sufficient unto themselves; when our merest cry called the comforting body to us, when it seemed that our urgency and anguish had the power to command the world. And now the loss of all this blamed upon the woman's body, which has taught us our first terrible lesson in woman's independence, her subjectivity, her refusal to come when we call, her peculiar willfulness, her insistence upon leaving us crying there, the pin sticking, the diaper growing cold, the covers turned back, the wind blowing, the hours passing as we lie alone, screeching in darkness.

Ernest Becker describes this primordial experience of terror as the principal determining event in the childhood of this culture.

> In the face of the terror of the world, the miracle of creation, the crushing power of reality, not even the tiger has secure and limitless power, much less the child. His world is a transcendent mystery; even the parents to whom he relates in a natural and secure dependency are primary miracles. How else could they appear? The mother is the first and awesome miracle that haunts the child his whole life, whether he lives within her powerful aura or rebels against it. The superordinancy of his world intrudes upon him in the form of fantastic faces smiling up close through gaping teeth, rolling eerie eyes, piercing him from afar with burning and threatening glances. He lives in a world of flesh and blood Kwakiutl masks that mock his self-sufficiency. The only way he could securely oppose them would be to know that he is as godlike as they.[5]

And so we understand finally how we, as adult humans in this culture, have acquired a certain anxiety in the face of existence, this dread that our modern psychologists and existential philosophers bring to the center of their discussion of the human being's position in this world.

But to their understanding we must add a further awareness, a sense of how our first struggle for control against the terror of the world, our first magical and realistic efforts to master the world and make it serve our need, was focused upon a woman's body. Thus, the abstract and philosophical issues as to the world's fundamental nature—its reliability, trustworthiness, or fundamentally treacherous being—were once very concrete and were learned in response to the presence or absence of a mother's body. Our very ambivalence toward existence reflects our ambivalence toward our mother's power. Philosophy is rooted in the first experience of a woman's flesh.

With this insight we begin to understand just how much we have invested in the way a woman appears and moves through the world and reaches out to touch us and lies down in bed with us; she who carries a primordial danger in her body, the power to take us back to this first crisis in our existential life.

When we attempt to determine the size and shape of a woman's body, instructing it to avoid its largeness and softness and roundness and girth, we are driven by the desire to expunge the memory of the primordial mother who ruled over our childhood with her inscrutable power over life and death. And we are driven by the longing to erase the past when we decide to impose our will upon a woman's body, inventing an ideal slenderness that will spare us a confrontation with whatever reminds us of the helplessness of our infancy. Above all, in an age when woman asserts her right to autonomy and power, we may be driven to evolve a cultural ideal that will release us from the dangers of remembering.

We know now what the fat woman, making her way past us in the supermarket, really means to us, what sort of symbolism and evocative power she carries in the sheer magnitude of her body. And we understand why we laugh at this woman, why we require this laughter to disguise our longing and our terror, why we refuse to sit on the seat where she sat and why, finally, we place her in scorn at the top of the fun house and forget the real meaning of this symbol. For beyond even the scorn she draws to herself, the fat woman is there as a reminder that we, too, once laughed and lived in the arms of a large woman, as if life were a place of transforming mirrors, everything we saw reflecting us back to ourselves, and this world a place of pleasure, of uninhibited delight, presided over by a woman's laughter.

13. BOY AND GIRL

At birth it's normal to find milk seeping from the baby's nipples, both males' and females'. (It used to be called witch's milk.)
—Nissa Simon

In Arabian religion a god and goddess were paired, the goddess being supreme, the god, her son, a lesser deity. Gradually there was a change whereby the attributes of the goddess were presented to the god, thus lowering the position of the female below the male.
—H. Robertson-Smith

Discovery consists of seeing what everybody has seen, and thinking what nobody has thought. —Albert Szent-Györgyi

WE HAVE GONE BACK, we have entered childhood again and imagined what it might be like to come to consciousness in the arms of a woman. This central fact of our existence, as it prevails almost universally in this culture, helps us to account for so many of the ambiguities in the relations between women and men. It gives us a sense, too, that we understand the urgency and obsession with a woman's body that is a predominant fact of our lives. If we place pornography and the tyranny of slenderness alongside one another we have the two most significant obsessions of our culture, and both of them focused upon a woman's body.

Indeed, from the primordial experience to which we have just returned we can now derive a far deeper understanding of much that we have observed so far. We are in a position, finally, to understand why girls are inclined to develop an obsession with their own bodies and attempt to starve and change them and make them smaller than they are by nature, while boys make the body of woman the scapegoat for their complex sufferings over all the ambiguities and difficulties of existence.

We can understand, also, the suffering of that unfortunate and depressed man who wrote to Dear Abby, so desperately concerned to control the body of his wife. We understand the terrible ambivalence that has caused him to suffer over his wife's larger size. We know why he was particularly troubled when she grew larger after childbirth and became a mother, why he felt the necessity to punish and threaten her, and why he was driven to leave her.

And we can finally understand the origins of a male envy of a woman's body, which plays such a large part in the masculine desire to keep women out of positions of authority and power.

For consider: the boy and girl grow older, they leave infancy and they leave behind in what is called the unconscious (that great unresting realm of significant memory) this entire time of life when woman was all-powerful. Growing up, they move into the social world and encounter the father and the world of the father. Now they drive away all memory of infancy if it attempts to return and draw them back into that seething, primordial swamp of an original ambivalence.

But the body awakens them with forgotten desires, breeds memory, brings the oldest struggles along with it, reminds us of the need to control it, the need to direct its urges toward appropriate places and objects. The body reminds them of their helplessness and recalls the oldest feelings of vulnerability we ever knew, waking alone and calling out for the body of woman in that first learning of the unforgivable terror.

But here we see how there is a parting of the way for girl and boy; how the boy, whenever anything in life threatens him with a feeling of being out of control, will turn to the body of woman to reassure himself and wish to take control over her body, the way he wished also in his earliest childhood. But now his obsession will take a sexual form, in keeping with the time of his life and the expectations of his culture. Even this sexual urge, which seems to belong so exclusively to instinct and nature, can serve him in his purely human need to take absolute command over a woman's body, which stands for all that is inscrutable, unpredictable, and uncertain in life. When he feels helpless or vulnerable, whenever there is a crisis in his life, he will wish to approach this body from a position of power, insisting upon his conjugal rights over it, legislating these, taking, having, possessing this body, making it, making it surrender, making it belong to him, laying it, as he himself was taken up and made safe and laid upon the breast of woman, belonging to her, her son, her infant, her child, possessed then with joy and comfort, and possessed also with terror and fear. It is called a reversal; for now, in his relations with women, he has been able to return to his first experience of being out of control and needing a woman's body. But now he is in a position of power.

Yet we know that his efforts to take command over woman's body are not limited to his sexual relations with women. We can imagine that a man, who was once helpless and dependent upon a woman's body, would be eager to develop an order of civilization in which he, and not woman, possessed power and authority. We can understand how he would value a social system in which woman was kept helpless and was made dependent upon him, in which her devotion to him was therefore ensured, in which it was guaranteed that her body would be available exclusively to him. In pursuit of this highly desirable situation he might be tempted to deprive her of money, and independence, and subjectivity, so that she could not threaten him with a return to that childhood situation he has escaped precisely through the creation of a world in which woman has become an object. Indeed, in this world of his own making he can live out again and again his oldest obsession with a woman's body, but now from a position of power—paying for that body when he has need, purchasing this body through his offer of social position and security, locking this body into the home and family he creates in order to be sure that this body will be there exactly when he needs it.

We can imagine how a man would wish to improve upon even that measure of control his social system gives him over a woman's body, would create culture and make pictures of this body that provide him with a woman's presence whenever he wishes for it, so that he now commands his own urgency, forcing the woman to come to him whenever he turns the pages of the book or the calendar, and shaping this body to the exact measure of his desire, large or small to his liking, and if her breasts are big and her hips round and full, making certain that in the picture she is now bound and chained and gagged and helpless—these pornographic images with which patriarchal culture soothes its own terrors of woman. And we can imagine how, in the ideal images he shapes of a woman's body—the images that will help him impress upon woman the way his culture wants her to look—he will be tempted to inflict upon her body all the resentment he feels because he is not woman, primordial goddess. For now he secretly longs to strip from her all this power she has been given by her natural condition. And so he, multiplied by the billions, creates an ideal image of woman in which she is not yet woman—is unripe, sometimes childlike, the breasts small and undeveloped, the hips narrow, the thighs slim, the shoulders slender. The anorexic girl steps forth. It is an image purged of the power to conjure up memories of the past, of all that could remind us of woman's mysterious power.

Thus, we can observe this ideal woman he has created to wear the fur coats he puts upon her shoulders—this woman, a symbol of his power, to whom he offers his arm as she steps from the car. She is adorned with the jewelry he has given her, her long, slender leg reaches out and is visible now through the slit in the narrow dress, which defines her angularity and her obedience to his requirements for her body. For here we can discover just how important the control over the body of a woman would be to a man. If he can persuade her to abandon the natural inclination of her own flesh, to reduce its size, starve it of its natural power, make its roundness lean and its curves angular, he will have succeeded in imposing his will upon everything the woman's body represents—universe and life, nature, fate and destiny, what is awesome and mysterious, capricious, uncontrollable, subjective and willful and has power over his life and death. This ideal image he forges of woman, which seems at first sight the least of his undertakings in this struggle to subdue woman, to guarantee her availability, to strip her of her power according to nature, and ensure that he does not ever recall it, contains in fact all these other social and sexual and existential strivings and is symbolic of his entire struggle to master his need for and fear of woman, around which his culture, his civilization, and his social system have been built.

"Would anyone care to learn something about the way in which ideals are manufactured? Does anyone have the nerve?"

But what of us, we women of this culture, who have accepted this ideal? If we have begun to live out our lives within these bodies as if they were enemies, struggling against them, inflicting penances upon them, subjecting them to extremes and rigors which might have done justice to a desert saint, how much, indeed, this tells us about the way in which we approach this same fundamental task of coming to terms with what is problematic and uncontrollable in existence—how we deal with the same primordial experience of being helpless and out of control and anxious and impotent and dependent. For us, there is no necessity to create a subservient class of human beings in order to deal with the rage and fear of primordial abandonment. For us, as women, the opportunity exists to come to terms with this essential crisis of existence by turning to our own bodies, made in the image of our mother's body and representing to us, as hers did in childhood, life and nature, fate, destiny, universe and uncontrollable world.

Here we recall the anorexic girl who said: "To have control over your body becomes an extreme accomplishment. You make of your body your very own kingdom where you are the tyrant, the absolute dictator."[1] Now we understand the supreme significance of these words: through them, the girl has revealed the most hidden strategy of the urge to starve the flesh. For in this kingdom of the body, where we have become the tyrant and absolute dictator, the childhood situation can be reversed, as neatly and precisely as it was for the man taking possession of a woman's body, when his entire culture makes certain it must be surrendered to him.

We know how easy it is to move between the body and the world—this body which was once all the world to us. Now, let us say, the faucet is leaking, it is impossible to find someone to repair it, and our anxiety grows because everything is getting out of control. The way the plants look reflects this, too, our attention focusing suddenly on everything that is worm-eaten and snail-bitten and growing to seed, and now also the cracks that have developed in the plaster since the last earthquake, the amber stains along the ceiling where the rain leaked in—all these ominous suggestions that this house that contains us and keeps us safe is under siege, breaking down, and there is no one coming to help us. Soon, going back and forth between the telephone and the window, a sense begins to grow that we are eating too much, nibbling a bite of cracker, talking to neighbors, munching on a cracker, making calls for repairmen, breaking off a piece of stale Oreo cookie, as if it were our appetite that were leaking, the careful control over the body which was cracking, one's own flesh going to seed. One feels ungainly, bustling about in the kitchen, and now we begin to remember that large meal eaten the week before. It seemed tolerable at the time but clearly, upon reflection, it must have put on pounds. For these pounds are now suddenly visible. We pinch our waist, it is decidedly softer; a quick glance down at the ankles confirms this impression of gathering bulk. And now, as the anxiety grows, and is focused upon the body, it seems that an immense hunger is growing, too, a longing to take everything in the world and put it in the mouth. We are standing, in fact, in front of the refrigerator. And indeed, our hand is reaching out. . . .

Thus, it happens that within an hour or two we have eaten what surely must be too much food. We have confirmed ourselves in the impression that it was our bodies that were getting out of control. And we have convinced ourselves, with a last, anguished glance in the mirror, that we have indeed gained weight. Our anxiety has shifted from the house to the body; it has moved from a world which has proved uncontrollable to a body which will surrender to governance—a new diet on the following day, a rigorous regime of exercise.

Our obsession is, at heart, an attempt to solve this primordial terror, which an entire school of modern thinkers has described as fundamental to our existence. For all its seeming triviality, this compulsive urge to reduce the size of the body is nothing less than a struggle to gain control over a universe that threatens us with abandonment and annihilation. In the face of this danger we direct our attention toward a woman's body, as we did already in our earliest childhood. In our relationship now to our own flesh we live out our yearning for omnipotence, our longing to control the world, our need to control the body of our mother and to have power over it. Through our obsession we are enabled daily to return to the original childhood situation, but now (we hope) from a position of power.

The equation is exact and precise: if the mind once longed for power over a woman's body as we lay wailing in darkness, this power we can now take over our own body. We can make it look the way we wish it to look, change its shape, control its natural urgings, conquer these, maybe even eliminate them. In this way, too, the mind can prove its command over existence, over material reality, over the nature that lives in the body. We can now grow imperious towards our appetites and subject them to starvation. We can become superior to the bulges in our flesh and drive them into angularity. However hard this struggle against the body might be, it is easier than to take command over the elusiveness of existence, the capriciousness of life, the sudden appearance of unexpected tragedies, unknown fate, uncontrollable destiny. "My stomach," says the anorexic girl, "is an inevitable fate."

And we see: yes, although she speaks this with despair, it is much easier for her to make her body represent the world and become her kingdom, where she is the tyrant, the absolute dictator, than to become in fact tyrant and dictator of an entire world.

For here we come upon the most troubling aspect of our obsession—this opportunity it gives us to express towards our own flesh whatever angers we have acquired toward woman, our mother, throughout our life. The rage of the breast withdrawn when we wished to suck it, the rage of the cover thrown back and the diaper growing cold, the rage of the child compelled to renounce her body's pleasures. The mother insisting upon this renunciation, not permitting the child to touch herself in private places, forcing the child to confine her eliminations to a place behind closed doors. The mother, who is herself, perhaps, not wholeheartedly in agreement with these stringent requirements of patriarchal civilization, now instructing her daughter in her social position, how she is not to run wild and shout and walk on the edge of a high wall like her brother. This rage, at the narrowing of possibility, the circumscription of her being, the little dresses that must be kept clean, the white blouse that must not become smudged, and he is climbing a tree and picking up stones and putting them in his pocket, while mother looks on with pride at his mud-splattered shoes, holding them up for everyone to see, this sign of his virility in the world. And the anger of separation from the mother, at this body once so close and now withheld; the growing knowledge, as the girl becomes adolescent, that she, unlike her brother, will never again be allowed to turn to this woman's body for comfort and relief from her struggles in the world. All the random and all the unreasonable rages the girl is encouraged by her culture to feel against her own mother—because she is older than other mothers, works when they do not or doesn't work and has a college education she doesn't use, speaks with a foreign accent, seems too American and middle-class. And there is the struggle to separate from her and not to identify with her, the longing to be just like her, the need to transcend the limitations of her life, and the guilt at this longing for transcendence, the rage at this complexity of feeling, the ambivalence, the ambiguity, the issues of merging, the losing of self in the love of the mother, and the enforced renunciation of this love.

Now all these rages can be directed by the girl at her own body. If men are cruel to women, or withholding, or rape us, and make pictures of us in which we are being tortured and abused, and become sadistic to women as an expression of rage against the mother, we as women are spared the temptation to inflict this torment upon another human being. Our own bodies will serve to receive the rage we would like to direct against our mothers.

And so we create a hell for the body, in which it can be afflicted with all the torments pornography inflicts upon the body of woman, the same sufferings our mythology reserves for sinners in the underworld. Thus, the female body is starved, emaciated, bound, driven, tortured with cold, shaken by rubber belts, forced to run on rubber treadmills going nowhere in their eternal pointlessness. This body is punished the way Tantalus was for his crime of eating the immortal nectar of the gods. Food is withdrawn as the mouth reaches out for it. Liquid withheld as we reach out to sip. The body is made to lift weights too heavy for the back to bear. In our ascetic striving for a slenderness that can never be achieved, we become like Sisyphus, eternal toilers at a task that, at the moment of its accomplishment, always seems to reverse itself, the pounds come on again, the conquered appetite returns, the rock rolls down the hill, and tomorrow the futile toiling must begin again.

Compulsive dieting is based upon the principle of reversal. If we once felt helpless, when it was we who hungered and waited to be fed, now it is we who make these crucial decisions as to the granting or withholding of what the body needs. But what an extraordinary feeling of power the act of dieting brings to us, as we refuse to grant the body's request to eat. Hour after hour, day after day, we watch it endure its growing hunger, knowing that now it is we who can decide when this torment will come to an end.

Compulsive dieting repeats over and over again the childhood situation, in the hope that we can at last master the dread and terror we once felt. If we are tempted finally to drive this situation to its furthest extreme; if we seem determined in our emaciation virtually to starve the body to death, we understand how the ultimate reversal of the childhood dilemma requires that we must take up, through our own bodies, the power over life and death.

For this is what fascinated us as we stared at the hunger artist in her golden cage. When the torches were lit and the wind came blowing, and we watched her shivering there in her meager straw, what we observed was the enactment of the ancient drama of her infancy, in all the profound horror of its reversal. For now as she holds out towards us this emaciated arm over which she has expressed her will, we see that this arm is indistinguishable from the arm of her mother; we understand that this body of hers, which is growing feeble and is wracked with the longing for food, is both her own infant body, subjected now to her own will, and the body of her mother, subjected to the torment that expresses the girl's unconfessed, unacknowledged, and unforgiving rage.

Thus, we understand, at last, why it is that we, as women, permit our culture to make us, through our bodies, the scapegoat for its suffering over the difficulties of existence. Women and men together we have early learnt to blame the body of woman. Together, we have raged against it and yearned for it, been tormented by its absence, stood in mortal need of its closeness, thought of it as fate, felt it as destiny, and knew it to be world.

Of course we allow ourselves to become our culture's scapegoat: we share with our culture a rage toward woman. Naturally, we cannot resist the statements it makes of uneasiness and hostility toward the flesh; we too have learned this hostility during the prolonged primordial moment, as we grew to consciousness on our mother's flesh.

For here, finally, is the meeting place toward which we have been wending our way, where culture and psyche converge; where the original infantile ambivalence is implanted in the structure of the mind, which one day will give rise to culture as an expression of its dilemmas. We are the scapegoat because the men of our culture blame their mothers. We permit them to direct this blame towards us because we, too, share this hatred —this hostility and ambivalence towards the feminine.

In this light we should be able to look at the adolescence of a growing girl in a new way. For at this moment in her development the entire host of charged and contradictory feeling must come on her, unavoidably now, when it is from her own chest that the breasts grow, from her own flat stomach that the rounded belly emerges, from the angular line of her hip and thigh that the rounding hips and swelling thigh of her mother now appears. One can imagine the terror of this re-emergence (which the boy is spared). We can appreciate how the girl might be driven to make this body reverse its natural tendency to look like her mother. We understand why she might be tempted to make it retreat from what is happening to it—to drive away the breasts and flatten the stomach and make angular the hip, in order to keep the body from acquiring the capacity to breed memory and awaken ambivalence. In adolescence the old, unresting infantile rage at the mother confronts the girl unavoidably, with the coming of her mother's body to the girl's own flesh.

But now, before we forgive our culture too easily for our sufferings over the body; before we let it go scot-free in this matter of our obsessive striving to conquer the body, let us examine the way in which our culture, in fact, fails us here. For we can imagine how much the mediations of culture could mean to the adolescent girl at this moment of crisis. Culture could assure her that it values her precisely for the feminine emerging now in her body and admires the power of the feminine and finds meaning in its relationship with nature. Indeed, if culture could welcome her into positions of prestige and authority because her body now shows that a girl has become woman; if it could help her through this transition, offering her a rite of passage in which she read to her community from its holy books and took the place of the rabbi and was respected by the congregation, she might pass through this crisis of ambivalence and come to regard her body with the original delight she took in woman's body, remembering not only her terror and rage, but recalling all those hours and months and years of rapt vision she shared with the infant Stieglitz, and remembering with pleasure the all-powerful status of her mother, which she now, too, would be welcomed to share.

For at that moment when her body is maturing and comes to remind her of her mother's body, something might happen to a girl that could transform her entire experience of living in a body. If the association between her mother and her self were positive, if her mother were a being of power and force, if that force were admired, if women were held in esteem for being women, the coming of maturity to the adolescent body of a girl would be a wonderful opportunity for her to transform the negative aspects of the original childhood experience of the body. She would thus be able to set aside her struggle against it and come to admire the female body instead. Indeed, through this experience she might forgive the body for all its childhood betrayals and defeats of her will, for its vulnerability, its slowness in learning, its dependency upon others, its resistance to the ambitions of the mind. Now, ripening into womanhood, the girl might learn that the whole sphere of sensual existence was as dignified and worthy as the assertion of self through mind. She might even be able, through this new, positive experience of the body, to forgive the mother of her childhood. Her adolescence would become a time of reconciliations.

Indeed, nature and the body's own dynamic transformations could perform for the adolescent girl a profoundly healing service even in a culture that cannot manage to grant to women a full political and social equality—if only culture managed not to interfere. This sacred drama unfolding between a girl and her body can be found in the life of Anne Frank, who spent the formative years of her adolescence hidden away from the world in her secret annex.

> I think what is happening to me is so wonderful . . . and not only what can be seen on my body, but all that is taking place inside. . . . Each time I have a period—and that has only been three times —I have the feeling that in spite of all the pain, unpleasantness, and nastiness, I have a sweet secret, and that is why, although it is nothing but a nuisance to me in a way, I always long for the time that I shall feel that secret within me again.[2]

Anne Frank experienced a sense of shame that made it impossible for her to speak of these new feelings and sensations. But she confided them to her diary. "Sometimes," she wrote, "when I lie in bed at night, I have a terrible desire to feel my breasts and to listen to the quiet rhythmic beat of my heart."

The genius of this girl, which is so abundantly apparent in the way she writes, is evident also in how carefully, candidly and perceptively she observes herself. And therefore, from her, we can learn about a process of curiosity and forgiveness, an overcoming of shame through fascination, which brings her to a deeper reconciliation with her body than has been possible for most of us.

> I already had these kinds of feelings subconsciously before I came here, because I remember that once when I slept with a girl friend I had a strong desire to kiss her, and that I did so. I could not help being terribly inquisitive over her body, for she had always kept it hidden from me. I asked her whether, as proof of our friendship, we should feel one another's breasts, but she refused.[3]

Anne Frank is here experiencing a natural and healing curiosity, which has the capacity to influence profoundly a girl's relationship to the female body by awakening in her the old awe and reverence of her infancy. "I go into ecstasies every time I see the naked figure of a woman, such as Venus, for example. It strikes me so wonderful and exquisite that I have difficulty in stopping the tears rolling down my cheeks."

Adolescent girls are drawn to study their own reflection in the mirror. This musing observation of self becomes for them a ritual activity, performed in private, away from the judgmental, censorious, often punitive attitudes of their culture. It is a tender activity, having less to do with vanity, more to do with introspection and the acquisition of self-knowledge. "I saw my face in the mirror," wrote Anne Frank, "and it looks quite different. My eyes look so clear and deep, my cheeks are pink—which they haven't been for weeks—my mouth is much softer. . . ."

Every woman recalls the time—the first embarrassed, fascinated confrontation with the new self one is becoming. We can imagine this same moment in a woman of our own generation; in the wife, let us say, of the man who signed himself Depressed. We picture her, a girl like Anne Frank, as she looks admiringly at herself in the mirror. She is studying those breasts, that rounding belly, those fuller thighs that make her like her mother; her body is entering its rite of passage and through it she will soon be initiated into womanhood. It is a rare moment and it fills her with a strange and mysterious delight. She combs back her hair and puts a flower in it; she takes her mother's lipstick from the drawer and heightens the color in her cheeks. Now she is wearing perfume, she has draped a scarf across her, letting it fall down from her shoulders, and she dances now, her arms reaching up, her belly twisting. She has never seen this dance before but her body knows its motion, as one day it will know how to make a mother, and will guide her in knowledge of tenderness in the care of a child, this body bending itself now, no longer seeking to know itself through studying its reflection, but gathering directly a knowledge of its own force, its sensual power in the dance.

But now suddenly, the door opens and the girl turns, startled and delighted, afraid of what she senses must have been a transgression and yet still eager to share this new knowledge of delight discovered in the body. She stretches out her arms, dancing still, a smile on her lips, as in her innocence she steps toward him. It is her older brother, her father, an uncle who has been spending a weekend with the family. And he, misunderstanding, reaches out for her, transforming her innocent delight into seduction. Or he takes alarm and flings back over his shoulder as he retreats some ambiguous expression that makes her feel ashamed. Or he grows angry, snatches up a towel, throws it over her, as if this flesh discovering itself were an object of danger or disgust. Or maybe he flails out wildly, overcome all in the same moment by the desire and fear and rage of his own awakened primordial memory. He slaps her, shakes her by the shoulders, calls for her mother and sends her in to lecture the girl.

In this moment, culture has just intruded upon nature, upon a girl who, a moment before, in private, in a rare solitude, had glimpsed the natural and now lost possibility of reconciliation with the flesh.

We can imagine further how vulnerable this girl will be when she becomes a woman. We know how she will be sensitive to the response her husband makes to her body. We know what terrible shame she will endure when he writes to Dear Abby. She is a person whose cultural and personal experience reinforces only one side of the original childhood ambivalence. Indeed, her culture is forever reminding her how dangerous her body is. It calls the flesh a prison of adipose tissue, floods the marketplace with books and sermons, tells parables, asks God to take her away and thanks God daily that it was not made woman. It writes letters to newspapers about her, tells her to stay on her diet, makes images of its ideal woman, develops fashions, makes clothes too small for her and produces thousands upon thousands of pictures of bound women with large breasts and round hips. And therefore, we can understand how she might be supremely tempted to forget that there was ever beauty and power in the large body of woman; we see how she might come to know a fear, greater even than in childhood, of the female body that is taking possession of her girlish slenderness. We know why she might wish to drive it away and keep it from developing and retreat from the complexity of associations her body carries with it. Oh yes, we comprehend now why she becomes obsessed.

We can imagine further what it means to this girl, confronted with the coming of her own womanhood to her body, that the round shape of her mother is never seen in a position of power or respect, that this roundness is only seen serving dinners and this abundance is only known clearing up dishes, and this fullness is only encountered telling people to wear their galoshes. That in our culture roundness rarely speaks in a poetic voice, abundance does not philosophize nor fullness speculate about the meaning of existence; that it cleans the toilet and nags the children and pesters the husband. And that, although the labor of what is round might be intrinsically graceful, it has been defined as the epitome of gracelessness, until the body of the mother comes to mean to the adolescent girl observing her mother nothing but matron, shrew, or drudge.

What a fateful collaboration there is between an original childhood ambivalence and a social system and a family structure that reflect this childhood situation, attempting in every way imaginable to reverse it at the expense of woman.

We can see also why the obsession with the body would emerge at that particular moment in the life of a people when its women were asserting their right to power and development, reclaiming the imagery of the Amazon, and threatening to restore to woman something of her original majesty and grandeur, her proud kinship with nature and her large size. We can understand how a man, unresolved in his ambivalence, afraid to confront again his original helplessness and dependency upon woman, would prefer to encounter a young girl than to confront this new woman of abundance who is emerging from the culture of her diminishment. We can understand how, in a frenzy of terror and dread, he might be tempted to spin out fashionable images of her that tell her implicitly that she is unacceptable to culture when she is large; and we can appreciate too how, faced with this call to our own development, asked to examine our complex history of relationship to women, to our mothers, to the feminine, we as women might also wish to retreat, and reduce the feminine in ourselves, confine it and subdue it, as it expresses itself through natural appetite and flesh. The wonder is that any of us know how to become women, or learn to delight in the coming of our mother to our body, and celebrate the fact that we too know how to bleed and heal ourselves, and produce food from ourselves and carry in our body the mystery of the conception of life. It is truly a wonder that any of us know how to take delight in our body's urges, welcome its hungers and cravings, delight in its sexual powers, surrender to its appetites. It is a wonder we don't all retreat from being woman and seek to starve ourselves, and refuse to become orgasmic, and dislike the emotionality in ourselves, and despise our intuitive gifts and perceptions, and despair over our similarity to animals and nature, and wear girdles and tight pants that restrict us, and adapt ourselves to the fashions, and conquer our bodies, and accept the warfare against it, and long to look like adolescent girls.

Whatever sympathy we feel for the adolescent boy, whose bodily urges are reminding him of a childhood situation he would rather forget, our heart must be wrung even more by the dilemma of the adolescent girl, who is asked in this moment of her development to become what her mother is—not by nature, but in all the restrictions imposed upon her by culture. For the adolescent girl is being brought by nature to become a woman, when everything in her culture tells her that woman is to be despised and feared.

14. THE MYSTERIOUS CASE OF ELLEN WEST

You must remember that a woman, by nature, needs much less to feed upon than a man, a few emotions and she is satisfied.
—Alice James

In our family group girls seem scarcely to have had a chance. . . . [Alice's] tragic health was, in a manner, the only solution for her of the practical problem of life. —Henry James

So much of the trouble is because I am a woman. To me it seems a very terrible thing to be a woman.
—Ruth Benedict

A WOMAN is riding; slowly now, her horse high stepping, his head high as she moves out along the gravel path of the park. Now she is well past the people strolling, the small girl playing around her governess on the park bench, the sound even of voices from the cafe where, beneath striped umbrellas, leaning out to watch her, eyes shaded, heads turning, someone must have been speaking her name and someone else remarking, not for the first time, how she, a woman, wearing men's clothes, was out riding alone.

Then, as the path begins to widen at the edge of the woods, and the trees grow more thickly clustering at the edge of the path, she gives her horse a freer rein, her shoulders relax imperceptibly, as if she is reluctant to admit her tension even to herself. Now her head is suddenly flung back. She is laughing, her right hand pressed against her heart, her shoulders shaking. It is the laughter of a girl carefree, beyond constraint, who in the next moment perhaps will begin to weep, totally given over to these waves of feeling, this ecstasy of freedom, her defiance, her soaring love for the bird passing so close to her face she can feel the feathering of air against her cheek. And she is riding.

She can imagine that the old woman gathering chestnuts beyond the last park bench is wondering how it is possible her father has let her learn to ride like a boy, and she presses her legs against her horse now, tightening her thighs; she removes her black cap and her hair, worn straight and much too short, falls down around her neck.

Ahead of her, flecked with a flickering dapple of sun and shade, just at the turning where the woods deepen and all suggestion of cultivated parkland is left behind, she glimpses the straight back, the perfect carriage of two riders; they are too far for her to be certain, but she is already galloping toward them, as if she knows who they are.

Now, anyone who sees her must be frightened for her; there is the worried frown of the old man coming from the woods, his book pressed tight between his hands at sight of these wild creatures—the horse with ears laid back, its eyes wide, suddenly tossing its head, tearing the reins from the rider, as the girl shouts out a challenge to those riders disappearing now among the trees. She is after them, bending low beneath the low branches, her eyes fiery, and the man calls out, the horse, he cries, is dangerous, however could they let her ride it, and the riders smiling softly to themselves, knowing she is young, too inexperienced a rider, ease their horses into a gallop.

Now she is no longer capable of thought; her legs closing, urging the horse forward, her head bent against his neck, the way no girl has ever been seen riding.

The path begins to narrow; ahead of her, clearly visible, the riders fall back one behind the other. She is riding toward them, not so much as glancing for a way to pass them through the woods, urging the horse forward, overtaking, and she hears the man cry out her name, she is edging him off the path, Ellen West, he calls, and she is passing the woman riding ahead, forcing her back against a tree, and again now, the way clear before her, the horse running with her own "terrible urge for freedom," her blood "racing and roaring," her breast "bursting" with power; and she knows, she knows, "this ardent yearning for a wild joy will not dry up." Not ever. But now as she rides out into a clearing in the woods, and pauses there, breathing heavily, the world recedes before her, and suddenly it seems to her that the "murmuring and rustling in the woods might be her dirge." Now, she longs for it to be night. She throws her hands over her face and cries out, smothering her words: "If thou still rulest behind clouds, Father, then I beseech thee, take me back to thee!"[1]

Her name was not Ellen West. That name was given to her by Ludwig Binswanger, the existential psychiatrist, when he wrote an account of her life in 1944, piecing it together from his research into her medical history, her own writings, and his direct experience with her. She had been treated some thirty years before the publication of his report, had been in analytical therapy and several times had hospitalized herself for help with severe depressions, suicidal thoughts, and a relentless obsession with eating and losing weight.

My interest in Ellen West dates back to the time when I first realized that in the story of her life we are presented with an incomparable parable. Hers is the story of a woman's struggle to live out her sensual nature, to live fully in her body and feelings, to find meaningful expression for herself, to find work and worthwhile activity in the world. For this girl has the qualities of which greatness is made: passion and vision, a wild ambition, a powerful social awareness, an overpowering thirst for learning and development, an impassioned love of life, a great gift for expression.

Ellen West failed in her struggle for self-development. She could not liberate herself from her culture's fear of women or from her own fear of her passionate nature. Yet, from the life of Ellen West it will be possible for us to learn how the failure of a woman's self-development inevitably becomes obsession. For that is the way Ellen West's story has taught me to regard our obsession—as a binding and yoking, as a subversion of the great creative power of woman in a futile struggle against nature and the body.

It is clear, from Binswanger's account, that Ellen West was growing up in the Europe of Bleuler and Freud, where she moved, at the age of ten, "from her original homeland." Thus, she grew to womanhood in a period of European history when women were seeking a greater freedom; and when fashions for women were shifting from the voluptuous to the more ascetic and slender, influenced no doubt by the same retreat from feminine power that inspires this change today. Unfortunately, however, we never learn Ellen's original homeland and we do not know the year of her birth. (Indeed, we do not even know exactly what she looked like, although one of her doctors described her as a woman of "medium height, adequately nourished, tending toward pyknic habitus, whose body build is characterized as boyish. The skull . . . large and massive. Facial form oval and evenly modeled.") Yet, the girl called Ellen West, who remains nameless, wearing a mask, has come in my mind to stand for all those women who have struggled for their development and failed, whether in her time or our own. Her life, with the vagueness of its biographical details, its unknown origins, its anonymity, suggests a mystery: why exactly did Ellen West become an obsessive instead of a woman fulfilled through some artistic expression or meaningful action in the social world?

The answer to this question must be looked for in the distinctive nature of Ellen's personality, and in the conventional nature of her family as well. For it is in this conflict between what she might have been, and what her family intended her to be, that the first clue to our mystery may be found.

As it happens, the father of Ellen West was a very wealthy man, externally self-controlled, stiffly formal and reserved. Although he was Jewish and lived in a time and place when anti-Semitism was a powerful social force, he was a "willful man of action," highly successful in the practical world. And yet he was, for all his active nature, internally soft and sensitive, "suffering from nocturnal depressions and states of fear accompanied by self-reproaches, 'as if a wave of fear closed over his head.' "

Ellen's mother is not described with the same detail. About her, we know only that she was a "soft, kindly, suggestible, nervous woman, who underwent a depression for three years during the time of her engagement" to Ellen's father.

But now, to these two people of the conventional, upper middle class, a passionate little girl is born; and she, from the first moments of her existence, shows highly distinctive traits. Thus, at the age of nine months she refuses to drink milk and can never again tolerate it. Later, as a small girl, she refuses to eat sweet desserts. We are told that she is a "lively, headstrong and violent" girl. We learn that one day, when she is shown a bird's nest, she insists that it is not a bird's nest and "nothing would make her change her mind."

Taken by themselves, without the testament of Ellen's life, we would have no reason to attach great significance to these details. But when we know of the obsession that follows, we shall be inclined to see in this cluster of disparate facts the very pattern which underlies the eventual development of obsession.

For instance: we may suspect that Ellen's father is a man in conflict and that this is precisely the reason we might give for his nocturnal depressions and fears. He is a man who lives a daytime and a nighttime existence, which are sharply divided from one another, presenting us with two faces, two personalities, a fundamental split. Indeed, some indication of the severity of this inward division can be seen in his two sons. For these boys seem to personify and to live out the two sides of their father's nature. The older, who "resembles his father," is well adjusted and cheerful, "without nerves." He appears to have been made to the measure of the older man's external self. But the younger has clearly been shaped by the father's inner, softer, more fearful nature. We are told about him that he is a "bundle of nerves, a soft and womanish aesthete."

The conflict that remains hidden in the father becomes visible in the next generation. We now have two sons, each of whom is half of what his father is; and we have a daughter who, in the beginning at least, remains whole. The conflict that is divided between her brothers she seems to have inherited directly. In her turbulent and troubled life, it is she who brings to fullest expression the conflict and self-division that are the outstanding characteristics of her family and its culture.

Indeed, when Ellen West grew up this conflict became dramatically apparent. Twice she fell in love and twice her father opposed her marriage, once to a "romantic foreigner" and once to a student for whom she felt an intense, passionate, and sensual attachment. From this, then, we may understand that Ellen's father felt some considerable ambivalence about passion, sensuality, and romance; and that this precisely was the essence of the conflict he passed on to his daughter.

Unfortunately, we cannot imagine that Ellen's mother would have been able to offer her daughter any model for successful rebellion or transcendence; her own longing for development, passion, and freedom must have been sacrificed for the sake of her marriage and experienced then only as a depression during the time of her engagement.

All this is indeed familiar. In the family of Ellen West we find a mother and father who bear the typical problems and dilemmas of their culture. And we can imagine that their passionate little daughter will early be impelled to protest against the feminine role these people expect her to fill.

Indeed, it is precisely in these terms that I interpret Ellen's early rejection of milk. For this, it seems to me, is a first, precocious rejection of the feminine, a turning away from that intimate, sensual relationship to the mother, which in this culture often promises such fateful social limitations for a girl.

But Ellen is above all precocious; she is a child whose earliest years contain, in a highly condensed, symbolic form, all the later issues of her childhood and life. Binswanger tells us that she once "confessed that even as a child she had passionately loved sweets"; and thus, he writes, her refusal of desserts was "clearly not a case of an aversion but probably an early act of renunciation." Here let us notice that what Ellen is in fact so precociously renouncing is her own earliest passion. She is following the pattern her father has set down for her. Already at this young age, along with the tendency to rebel, Ellen is showing an inclination to remain loyal to her father's choices.

But what shall we make of her contradictory utterance about the bird's nest? Can we see it as a protest against the conventional definitions of home and family that are being offered to this girl? For indeed, her statement is a violent opposition to the "nature of reality" as it is presented to her through these feminine symbols of nesting and homemaking and child-rearing. "This bird's nest is not a bird's nest," she says. And she means: I will not accept your vision of reality; I am a woman who will not accept this nest as destiny.

We should not be surprised that Ellen West begins this protest so early in life or that she is already in conflict over it. For we must recall that she has been born to a time and culture far more repressive of women than our own, and we shall soon learn that she is a being with an imperative need for all those things conventionally denied to a woman. She has a temperament entirely unsuited to what is expected of a girl, a nature that will make it very difficult for her to accept her destiny as her culture ordains it. This, I suggest, is one answer to the mystery of her life.

For Ellen West is a brilliant girl, an excellent student, highly ambitious; a girl "who weeps for hours if she does not rank first in a subject." She is of "lively temperament and still self-willed." She feels an "uncontrollable urge to freedom, as if she must achieve something great and mighty." She knows a "consuming thirst to learn," has a keen and vital social consciousness; "reads much, occupies herself intensively with social problems, feels deeply the contrast between her own social position and that of the 'masses,' and draws up plans for the improvement of the latter."

Consequently, we are not surprised to discover that she early adopts as her motto: *aut Caesar aut nihil* ("either a Caesar or nothing"). Of course she must choose a man as the ideal on which to model herself. What does her culture offer her by way of an image through which, as a woman, she can find greatness or success in the world? Inspired by such thirsts and ambitions, she is compelled to wish to be a boy. Thus, until she was sixteen years old, she "preferred to wear trousers" and played only at boys' games. Even in her seventeenth year, in a passionate poem of longing for life and fulfillment, "she still expressed the ardent desire to be a boy."

Ellen West displays what Binswanger calls a "marked variability of mood," this sense of being called to greatness, invariably followed by a feeling of dejection. From this we may imagine that the girl is enduring a great conflict, that she is filled with an ambition her culture will not approve of in a woman. Indeed she yearned ardently for work, both that she might fulfill herself and because she recognized that work might help her to resolve her conflicts. "When all the joints of the world threaten to fall apart," she wrote, "when the light of our happiness is extinguished and our pleasure in life lies wilting, only one thing saves us from madness: work."

This need to externalize her own struggles, to engage them through meaningful interaction with the world, cries out again and again in the life of Ellen West. "Pityingly," the psychiatrist tells us, "she looks down upon all her fine ideas and plans and closes her diary with the burning wish that they might one day transform themselves into deeds instead of merely useless words." This girl is longing to step meaningfully into life. And she knows herself that this is next to impossible for a woman. "I have not kept a diary for a long time, but today I must again take my notebook in hand; for in me there is such a turmoil and ferment that I must open a safety valve to avoid bursting out in wild excesses. It is really sad that I must translate all this force and urge to action into unheard words instead of powerful deeds. It is a pity of my young life, a sin to waste my sound mind. For what purpose did nature give me health and ambition? Surely not to stifle it and hold it down and let it languish in the chains of humdrum living, but to serve wretched humanity."

At this stage of her life, Ellen is not at all compliant. She is actively looking for work, studying, writing in her diary, and writing poetry. Now and later in her life she longs to set herself against whatever represses growth and limits freedom. "You realize that the existing social order is rotten," she says reproachfully to herself in her diary, "rotten down to the root, dirty and mean; but you do nothing to overthrow it." Thus she becomes aware of the conventional elements in her own nature. She cries out at them from the pages of her diary: "Do you actually preach making concessions? I will make no concessions!" "I want a revolution," she writes, "a great uprising to spread over the entire world and overthrow the whole social order." But over and over again Ellen fails to find the meaningful activity she is seeking. She is driven back again and again to these impassioned utterances which then close themselves between the pages of her diary, as she observes the true nature of those forces which hold her back: "The iron chains of commonplace life," she says, "the chains of conventionality, the chains of property and comfort, the chains of gratitude and consideration, and strongest of all, the chains of life."

This is a woman in conflict, divided within herself, a girl in boys' clothing, playing boys' games, dreaming dreams deemed suited only to a boy. If this conflict were not enough (this longing to act within a world that does not allow action to women), we discover also what a passionate girl is Ellen West, how her "heart beats with exultant joy," how she longs for the wind to "cool her burning brow," and now, when she runs against the wind "blindly, careless of custom or propriety, it is as if she were stepping out of a confining tomb, as if she were flying through the air with an uncontrollable urge to freedom." Yet, inevitably this elemental passion is followed by a "darkened sky," the "winds blowing weirdly," a fear that the "fresh marrow of life" will grow stale, "the ardent yearning for a wild joy" dry up, and she will be left "pining away bit by bit."

All her life she moves back and forth between strong feeling and a retreat from it; between her exuberant, elemental nature and her concessions to the conventional world. Thus, we come to understand why she "cultivates riding with an excessive intensity," the way she does everything else. She is desperately longing for some form in which to express this passion that rises in her soul. This girl has, as I have said, the qualities of greatness: passion and vision, a wild ambition, a powerful social awareness, an overpowering thirst for learning and development, an impassioned love of life, a great gift for expression. And all this trapped within the confines of a woman's body. We know there will be trouble here.

"Who," asks Virginia Woolf, "shall measure the heat and violence of the poet's heart when caught and tangled in a woman's body?"[2] These words, written of Shakespeare's sister, the imaginary "Judith," might just as well have been written of the real girl, Ellen West. When we hear of Judith Shakespeare that she "killed herself one winter's night and lies buried at some crossroads where the omnibuses now stop outside the Elephant and Castle," we can imagine that some such destiny must also await our own Ellen West, she who must likewise have been "crazed with the torture that her gift had put her to," when as a woman, she was unable to develop it.

This is how we come to know her—torn between her ambition and her awareness of the terrible obstacles she will have to overcome in the world; driven by passion, which terrifies her and from which she always retreats.

A few years later she will confide to her diary: "I am twenty-one years old and am supposed to be silent and grin like a puppet. I am no puppet. I am a human being with red blood and a woman with a quivering heart. And I cannot breathe in this atmosphere of hypocrisy and cowardice, and I mean to do something great and must get a little closer to my ideal, my proud ideal. Will it cost tears? Oh, what shall I do, how shall I manage it? It boils and pounds in me, it wants to burst the outer shell! Freedom! Revolution!"

When Ellen West was twenty years old, she made "her second trip overseas to nurse her older brother, who is very sick." At this time, we are told, she still takes "pleasure in eating and drinking," although "this is the last time she can eat unconcernedly." Thus, until her twentieth year Ellen West did not suffer from obsession. She warred within her soul, as an adolescent girl might; she struggled with her family, she feared madness, she longed to be delicate and ethereal, she longed for greatness, she kept a diary, she wrote poems, she dressed like a boy, she developed a social conscience, her heart opened with joy and closed in despair and again opened, for she was no puppet, this woman with such wild and passionate heart. But now, in her twentieth year, a number of things happen: her brother falls ill, she becomes engaged to a "romantic foreigner," her father breaks off this engagement. Returning home from this trip she stops in Sicily and writes a paper, "On the Woman's Calling." Now she still "loves life passionately, her pulse hammers out to her fingertips, and the world belongs to her." And yet, we are told, these weeks in Sicily are the "last of her happiness in life." Something has happened, which has made all this adolescent joy and passion move towards obsession. For along with the wild "contradictoriness of mood" that has long been typical of her, "something new emerges now, a definite dread—namely, a dread of getting fat."

Here, knowing what it means to suffer from this obsession, a tremor of foreboding must come over us. At this moment a terrible resolution has been sought for the fertile conflict in which she found herself as a girl. It is a fateful moment in her life; and from now, until her death, she will never be freed from obsession; she will struggle against it, she will find brief moments of reprieve, but increasingly now from day to day her life will narrow, her interests become confined, all her passionate striving will be limited, her ambitions reduced, her growth as a human being will cease and in place of all her other strivings and idealisms, she will develop the one, sole, obsessive ideal of becoming thin. From now on she will be more than ever torn by conflict, but now the terms of this conflict will have shifted from the real and vital issue of her own development, her liberation, to this symbolic and sterile issue of how large her body is and how much food she has managed not to eat.

She is only twenty years old, but we, who know this obsession, know that Ellen has failed. Now, unless some meaningful intervention occurs, some help in understanding the real nature of her "illness," her obsession can only grow worse and at last destroy her.

Unfortunately, Ellen West was never offered a meaningful understanding of her condition as a woman. In her diaries and journals she struggled to understand the meaning of her obsession, just as in her daily life, she struggled to free herself from it and to find meaningful work in the world. Although she is seriously depressed when she arrives home from Sicily, she comes out of her depression when "she makes preparations for the installation of children's reading-rooms on the American model." Later, she studies for the Matura, the final examination in secondary school, which would have qualified her for entrance to any university. "She gets up at five, rides for three hours, then has private lessons and works all afternoon and evening until late at night, with the help of black coffee and cold showers." Some time later she studies for and passes the teachers' examination, "in order to be able to audit courses at the University." During the summer she goes to study at an unnamed university town. She becomes engaged to a student. Her parents, however, demand a temporary separation. Ellen then goes to a "seaside resort, and here once again an especially severe "depression" sets in. . . . "She does everything to get just as thin as possible, takes long hikes and daily swallows thirty-six to forty-eight thyroid tablets. Consumed by homesickness, she begs her parents to let her return. She arrives completely emaciated, with trembling limbs, and drags herself through the summer in physical torment, but feels spiritually satisfied because she is thin. She has the feeling that she has found the key to her well-being."

Now this becomes the pattern of her life—a struggle to liberate herself from her conventional family, a struggle to engage meaningfully in the world, and a struggle simultaneously against the depressive and obsessive thoughts that inevitably arise when she moves towards this goal. Meanwhile, the obsession grows more and more powerful. There is despair, depression, breakdown; the engagement broken off, weight gained and lost constantly, an unpleasant love affair, a growing concern with her body weight, a growing longing to be thin, an obsessive longing for food. We hear about a suddenly awakened love for music, her falling in love with her cousin, we hear about her "hating her body and often beating it with her fists." She marries her cousin, hoping to get rid of her obsession; hoping, no doubt, that this choice of the conventional world will free her from her frantic struggle with her body. Unfortunately, Ellen was mistaken in this hope. As the years pass, her obsession grows more and more severe. Soon, she is taking sixty to seventy laxatives a night, she experiences "tortured vomiting and violent diarrhea, often accompanied by a weakness of the heart." She weighs only ninety-two pounds. She writes to her husband that "my thoughts are exclusively concerned with my body, my eating, my laxatives." And finally, one day on a hike with him, the confession bursts from her "that she is living her life only with a view to being able to remain thin, that she is subordinating every one of her actions to this end, and that this idea has gained a terrible power over her."

But this was the girl who wrote poetry, the girl longing for revolution, the girl active and engaged in social undertakings, the girl who studied, the girl who made her way back to the university, the girl in love with life, ecstatically involved with the Universe (this poet who might have been, for all we know, one of the great poets of our century). Can we doubt there is an immediate relationship between the withering away of these possibilities for self-development and the growth of her obsession? Ellen West saw what we must now begin to see. She wrote: "I felt that all inner development was ceasing, that all becoming and growing were being choked, because a single idea [her obsession] was filling my entire soul: and this idea something unspeakably ridiculous. My reason rebelled against it, and I attempted by will-power to drive this idea out. In vain. Too late—I could no longer free myself and longed now for liberation, for redemption which was to come to me through some method of healing. Thus I came to psychoanalysis."

Ellen West could have been saved by a correct understanding of her obsession. If only she could have understood why she and her whole culture feared female power and the full development of woman; if only she had known women like herself, someone to have encouraged her, someone whose example might have assured her that however bitter her struggle, some solution to it was yet possible and so was survival outside the restricting claims of her family.

Ellen is a woman for whom psychoanalytic understanding might have meant a great deal, if only psychoanalysis had formulated correctly the cultural and psychological dilemma of women. She is a person gifted with an ability for introspection. She was crying out for help.

One of her analysts, interpreting her condition according to the theories of Freud, discussed her problems with "anal-eroticism." But she was deeper in her understanding than her analyst. She wrote: "Perhaps I would find liberation if I could solve this puzzle: the connection between eating and longing. The anal-erotic connection is purely theoretical. It is completely incomprehensible to me." She is right: liberation for her could only be found through an understanding of the connection between eating and longing; by a correct naming of her terrible urge to eat as a frustrated craving for self-development.

However, she met no one who could help her in this quest for understanding. Another doctor felt that she was suffering from "severe obsessive neurosis combined with manic-depressive oscillations." He endeavored to persuade her that her dread of getting fat was a dread of "being fertilized, becoming pregnant." He, however, did not raise the issue of the nest, whose "reality" she had rejected already in childhood, nor did he encourage her to understand that her fear of pregnancy was an entirely warranted dread of losing what was meaningful to her in life—her freedom, her passion, her self-development.

These interpretations would have been particularly relevant to Ellen West, for she was, at one time during her marriage, as she herself confessed, "willing to renounce higher intellectuality" in order to become a mother. Indeed, in the early days of that marriage she "concerned herself ostentatiously with the household and the copying of recipes, especially in the presence of her younger brother's wife, who is a slim blonde." And so we appreciate anew how this issue of what a woman must sacrifice to be a "mother and wife" and to fulfill a conventional destiny must have meant to Ellen West, with her passionate aspirations. And we may deeply regret that a fuller understanding of her dilemma was never offered to her.

Now, as she continued to grow more and more ill, in spite of her repeated efforts to write, to study, to undertake social projects, the famous doctor Kraepelin was finally called in; he diagnosed "melancholia" and failed also to interpret her terrible depressions as a sign of a conflict she was not able to resolve.

Ellen hospitalized herself as her condition continued to grow more severe; but even in the clinic and finally in the sanatorium there were laxatives, a struggle not to eat, a greater and greater emaciation, an increasing narrowness of interest, a focusing of her great gifts and energies on the issue of body and food. Eventually, the famous Dr. Bleuler (a co-worker of Freud) was called in, and a foreign psychiatrist was also consulted about her ceaseless torment. "A progressive schizophrenic psychosis" was diagnosed and Ellen's husband was offered "very little hope." The foreign psychiatrist, however, disagreed with this diagnosis because there was, in Ellen, no evidence of intellectual impairment.

Ellen West says: "I am in prison and cannot get out. It does no good for the analyst to tell me that I myself place the armed men there, that they are theatrical figments and not real. TO ME THEY ARE VERY REAL."

The prison is real. The armed men are real. They are the unnamed social, cultural, and psychological forces with which this woman was struggling. And because they remained unnamed, they finally destroyed her.

Following this diagnosis Ellen decided to take her life in her own hands and leave the sanatorium. Her weight, at that time, was 104 pounds. We are told that on her trip home she was "very courageous." But that should not surprise us. All her life she showed this courageousness, always trying to overcome the obsession she struggled in solitude to understand. In vain. On the way home her symptoms only appear more strongly. The reunion with her relatives intensifies her illness. And we know, reading this, that the woman's life is running out. She is thirty-three years old. She has tried everything she can think of to free herself from obsession. She has written a "history of a neurosis." She has sought professional help. She has hospitalized herself. While in the hospital she has written poetry exploring her condition. Now, all else having failed, she returns once again to her family, feeling completely "incapable of dealing with life."

The closing words of Binswanger's account of Ellen West's life read like the final words of a parable: "On the third day of being home she is as if transformed. At breakfast she eats butter and sugar, at noon she eats so much that—for the first time in thirteen years—she is satisfied by her food and gets really full. At afternoon coffee she eats chocolate creams and Easter eggs. She takes a walk with her husband, reads poems by Rilke, Storm, Goethe, and Tennyson, is amused by the first chapter of Mark Twain's 'Christian Science,' is in a positively festive mood, and all heaviness seems to have fallen away from her. She writes letters, the last one a letter to the fellow patient to whom she had become so attached. In the evening she takes a lethal dose of poison, and on the following morning she is dead."

For Ellen West, Mental Patient and Suicide

Lethal poison: revenge
on a world of definitions
coiled in the bird's nest
swimming in the milk
you refused   getting yourself a name
for stubbornness
You   weaning yourself
striding in boy's clothes
dreaming of freedom
in the skirted parlor
of pre-war Europe
you   child and poet
delivered at birth
into enemy hands

I am not of your women!
the poet in you
could only choke
on hunger
shame and self-loathing
Every ounce of your female flesh
revolted you
they took you to clinics
for willed starvation
for dread of swollen breasts
and swollen belly
They analyzed you twice
committed you to Kreuzlingen
in Switzerland
Your husband
understood you so perfectly
he came with you everywhere

Ellen West, a non-Swiss—
your title in Binswanger's history—
Ellen, not-ski-ing the planes of the mountain

not-carving the frozen air
with your eager, longing breath
not-living for thirty years
the definitions
they had prepared for you
not-giving-in
though hunger haunted you
in a false and fatal form
O Ellen
I sift your life up out of their negatives

I read of you
in anger   you surrounded
by understanding, understood
to the brink of your throttled life
by parents, husband, the greatest doctors
in Kreuzlingen, in Switzerland
in the nineteen-twenties

you surrounded
by snow-peaks   by glaciers
by chocolate creams
and Easter eggs   the poems
of Goethe and Rilke   you
hungry for a forbidden life
guilty   starving   condemned

by a world of definitions

taking lethal poison
with a tranquil face

During a conversation with Kim Chernin in the summer of 1980, about Ellen West and the thesis of this book, I recalled and pulled out of my files this poem, written in 1971 and never published. I am glad to have it appear now, in this context, at Kim Chernin's request.

—ADRIENNE RICH *1971*

15. THE OBSESSION

> Everything agitates me, and I experience every agitation as a sensation of hunger, even if I have just eaten.
>
> —Ellen West

> Eating is symbolically associated with the most deeply felt human experiences, and thus expresses things that are sometimes difficult to articulate in everyday language.
>
> —Peter Farb and George Armelagos

> To become conscious of the body and its operation was to become conscious of the spirit. The individuation process, therefore, could also be observed in the body. . . . In that understanding lies the treatment and the possibility of healing.
>
> —Marion Woodman

I have often wished that Ellen West might have known the work of Anzia Yezierska, who became famous during the 1920s as a writer of the Jewish immigrant experience in America. The two women, for all the differences in the social class, had a great deal in common. Indeed, for all we know, Ellen's mysterious "original homeland" might have been that same Russian Poland from which Yezierska came. Certainly, both women were alive at the same time, both were Jewish, both were writers, and both were required to struggle for their self-development against the dominance of their father's authority, culture, and values. Yezierska succeeded in this struggle, Ellen did not. We can imagine, therefore, what it might have meant for Ellen if she had been able to read, in particular, these words: "It was his practical formula for . . . success which drove me to defy all sound advice—all reason and common sense—to forsake family, friends, do without sleep, without clothes, withdraw from the world, from life itself—to write."[1]

We have never been told what it was that made it possible for Yezierska to say in her own life, and through her fictional heroines, a direct "no" to the patriarchal authority that laid claim to a woman's obedience and compliance. Perhaps it was the fact that she was desperately poor and had early learned the struggle for survival? Perhaps that she was fighting with real hunger and not with the metaphor of hunger, whose nature mystified her? Her work is filled indeed with images of hunger—a young girl boarding the train on her way to college, bending over the side of the seat, pinching pieces from a loaf of bread, and glancing sideways in fear people might see how famished she is.

But Yezierska also understood hunger as a metaphor. Indeed, hunger as a symbol for all that lies unsatisfied in the heart and soul may well be the most typical and recurrent image in her entire work.

She writes: "Something cried dumb in me. I couldn't help it. I didn't know what it was I wanted. I only knew I wanted. I wanted. Like the hunger in the heart that never gets food."

Or, from another character: "How I was hungering to go to America after that."

Or again: "Like the hunger for bread was my hunger for love."

All the great, elemental passions, Yezierska understands and expresses through the metaphor of hunger. Sometimes it is a hunger for love or for all that America means to the girl in the shtetl; sometimes it is a hunger for life itself, for the fullness of existence. But most often in Yezierska's work it is the hunger for education and self-expression that lies unresting in the heart, driving her and most of the characters she writes about.

"His huge, stoop-shouldered body leaning forward—quivering with hunger to grasp the secret turnings of the 'little black hooks' that signified his name."

"The only compensation for the artist is the chance to feed hungry hearts."

"I want knowledge. How, like a starved thing in the dark, I'm driven to reach for it."

In her remarkable novel, *The Bread Givers,*[2] Yezierska created the character of Sara Smolinsky, who lives out the struggle for woman's self-development through the metaphor of hunger. In this way, as in so many others, she is a spiritual sister to Ellen West. There is the same expressive greatness in both of them, the same will to life, to elemental joy, and to the creation of self.

In the life of Sara Smolinsky, however, the forces that are assembled to oppose women's development reveal themselves in stark and naked form. Thus, when Sara was a child the best portions of food were reserved for her father while she and her sisters sat "trembling with hunger" as they waited for him to take the "top from the milk" and the fat from the soup. Even when Sara grows up and is going to school at night and practically starving as she works in a laundry to support herself, she finds out that in the public cafeteria men are given larger portions of meat than the women who come through the line.*

This preference for the male over the female in the novel is reflected in more traditional ways as well. It is the father's books that were deemed worthy to be brought from the old country when the mother's gefilte-fish pans were left behind. In the new world Sara and her sisters are forced to sleep in cramped and crowded bedrooms so that their father will be able to study day and night in a special room.

Consequently, Sara must struggle at one and the same time for food, for the dignity of a woman's values, for a room of her own, and for the books withheld from women in her culture. For her, the right to eat comes in this way to signify a woman's right to be and to become, which her father explicitly opposed. "Pfui on your education," he screams at her. "What's going to be your

*This novelistic detail reflects a social and political situation which remains true in our time as well. Even today in every part of the world where people hunger, women receive less food than men. Moreover, what food they do receive is consistently less nutritious. (L. Leghorn and M. Roodkowsky, "Who Really Starves?" *Women and World Hunger,* New York, 1977.)

end? A dried-up old maid? You think you can make over the world? You think millions of educated old maids like you could change the world one inch? Woe to America where women are let free like men."

The mother of Sara Smolinsky cannot take her daughter's side in the girl's momentous struggle for freedom and education. Yet once, after this renegade daughter defies her father and leaves home, her mother travels for hours in order to bring her daughter a jar of herring and a feather bed. When she arrives she throws her arms around her and kisses her "hungrily." But she must leave after only a few minutes so that her husband will not find out where she has gone. And still, in spite of this hunger, which drives her out in search of her daughter on a freezing night, she wishes to see her married rather than at college. Still, she urges her to set her studies aside and come to visit her instead.

Sara Smolinsky must go on alone, without understanding from her mother, without help or support from her father, misunderstood also by her sisters, who have brought her a wealthy suitor, whom she rejects. It is only later, when she returns to visit her family again after years and years of absence, that some reward for this struggle comes to her from her own mother, who is dying and who now chants out gratefully from her death bed: "God be praised I lived to see my daughter a teacherin."

It is at this moment in the story that something is said that transforms understanding. It is not a momentous saying and it might easily be missed if we were not already attuned to the complex meanings of food and eating. For now, the mother of Sara Smolinsky dies; the neighbors come in to wail and mourn over her body and one of the women speaks these words, which prove to be unforgettable. "Never," she says in praise of Sara's mother, "never did she allow herself a bite to eat but left-overs. . . ."

With this statement we appreciate the full meaning of female hunger—of all the spiritual and emotional strivings it includes and just how forbidden these are to a woman. When Sara Smolinsky, the teacherin, later cries out from that room of her own she finally achieves: "I, Sara Smolinsky, have done what I had set out to do," we are prepared to understand just how mightily a woman must hunger in order to fulfill her vocation. At last we see how this power of a woman struggling for development might well be the greatest power in the world.

But here we must ask a melancholy question. Recalling all the similarities there are between the girl called Ellen West and the character named Sara Smolinsky, we are compelled to wonder why one of them succeeded while the other failed. For Sara Smolinsky's success charts the passionate rise of Anzia Yezierska's life from the same impoverished beginnings and against identical cultural and parental pressures. Why then did Yezierska succeed in living with her hunger until she found appropriate spiritual nourishment, while Ellen West turned against her appetites and spent the better part of her adult existence attempting to suppress them?

The answer to this question is given over and over again in Yezierska's novel, which is filled with episodes of healing rage. Sara Smolinsky is a fighter. Her longing for freedom and development are not limited to impassioned utterances closed between the pages of a diary. They are transformed into outrage and this rage is not directed against her self. It is turned rather against everything that limits her development. She fights against her father, and she fights against the husbands of her sisters, and she fights the wealthy suitor who offers her everything that conventional society can conjure up by way of temptation, and she fights her loneliness and her pity for her mother, and she fights even the ravaging intensity of her own physical hunger. We are left then with the unavoidable impression that it is precisely her rage which frees her from the submission her mother and older sisters could not transcend; this rage spoken directly and clearly to her own father:

"My gall burst in me," she says. "For seventeen years I had

stood his preaching and his bullying. But now all the hammering hell that I had to listen to since I was born cracked in my brain. . . . Should I let him crush me as he crushed them? No."

It is this "no" I wish Ellen West might have read. For all her giftedness and greatness we cannot imagine her like this, in open rebellion against her father. That same rage which proved to be so liberating for Yezierska made an invalid of Ellen West. She, unlike Yezierska chose to direct her rage against her body and appetite rather than against the culture and family that limited her life choices. That is why she became an obsessive rather than a woman fulfilled through her capacity to act and to create.

Nevertheless, Ellen West has something essential to teach us. Her failure, which proved so tragic where her own life is concerned, should not blind us to the fact that she accomplished something remarkable through the self-investigation she pursued lifelong in her diaries. For me, indeed, Ellen West became a mirror image of my own struggle to understand obsession. Rage, I had learned, came into a woman's life when her life choices were severely limited. But I still could not understand why this rage, directed against the body, had such a formidable power to affect a woman's intellectual and spiritual growth.

The answer to this question emerged for me one day from a single passage in Ellen's diary. There she writes that her body "shares in all the stirrings of her soul." And I, reading this phrase, realized that Ellen West had forged a missing link. "My inner self," she writes, "is so closely connected with my body that the two form a unity and together constitute my I, my unlogical, nervous, individual I."

In this equation, what is done to the body will simultaneously be done to the soul. Consequently, at that very moment in a woman's life when she turns with rage against her body, she begins to attack also her "inner self" and the whole feeling side of her nature. Her rage, which arose initially because of the restrictions imposed upon her self-development, is now directed, through her body, at the "inner self" which hungers for its development. It is a costly and tragic reversal. Whatever chance the woman might have had to grow and to express herself will now have vanished. For her obsession with her body is, fundamentally, an expression of violence towards her soul.

Thus, we can understand in a new way the fact that Ellen West takes an inordinate amount of laxatives, sometimes sixty or seventy tablets a night; and the meaning also of the "tormented vomiting," the "violent diarrhea." She is making an effort to *purge* herself of all her old yearnings and ambitions and sensual pleasures; to *eliminate* that entire feeling aspect of self, that "inner being" she wrote of. And why? Precisely because Ellen West is a girl who cried out: I am afraid of myself. I am afraid of the feelings to which I am defenselessly delivered over every minute.

Similarly, when we hear that Ellen had "been saddened when she looked at herself in the mirror, hating her body and often beating it with her fists," we may understand that this girl is flailing out against her own soul and is attacking it for all the problems it has created for her, by alienating her from her family, by filling her with desires a girl should not have, and by creating aspirations for which she finds no authentic, creative outlet.

Thus, from Ellen West we learn how a young woman invariably rejects, along with the female body, the passionate, "feminine" side of her nature, from which her creative development would arise.

The reasons for this rejection are complex, as we have seen. Fear of the elemental nature of the woman's feeling and a desire to remain loyal to the family and its culture frequently inspire this choice. But there is a further reason that will become clear to us in the life of Ellen West. For we can imagine how a girl like Ellen would believe that power and success in the world are only to be gained by taking up a conquering, masterful position over the "inner self," with its wayward appetites and unpredictable urges. We understand the temptation she would feel, with her urge for work and involvement with the world, to accept the masculine model for these achievements, to prefer will and discipline, logic and rationality, over the surrender to her passions and appetites.

And yet for Ellen West (as for Yezierska and Marian MacAlpin and Sara Smolinsky) self-expression and meaningful work could only have been found through an ability to continue living in her feelings. In them lay all her greatness, from them arose her astonishing insight and articulate utterance, from them the prompting beyond the limitations of woman's life, out into the world.

But how could she have known this? Her whole culture has taught her to fear the power of these feelings; her family has tutored her well in this. How could she possibly have guessed that her effort to obey the masculine choices of her father would afflict her with obsession and progressively would dry up the source of her creative force?

If we interpret obsession in this way, as an effort to control or eliminate the passionate aspects of the self in order to gain the approval and the prerogatives of masculine culture, we can at last explain the whole host of mysterious spiritual sufferings that belong to obsession—all those peculiar sensations of emptiness, of longing and craving, of dread and despair from which we suffer.

For there is tragedy in our obsession; and not the least of this tragedy is the fact that the spiritual struggle in which we, as women, are engaged remains hidden by the apparently trivial preoccupations of our obsession. What might be seen as great and heroic in us, worthy of respect and admiration, is lost because we have as yet no universal language to discuss a woman's struggle for the soul.

Ellen West was struggling towards this language. Indeed, her earliest references to obsession include also a vivid expression of her spiritual condition. Thus, she writes that she has begun to feel herself "small and wholly forsaken in a world which she cannot understand." She writes that "she has no home anywhere," that "she does not find the activity she is seeking, that she has no peace, that she feels a veritable torment when she sits still, that every nerve in her quivers, and that in general her body shares in all the stirrings of her soul."

What Ellen West has here described is the suffering of a woman alienated from an essential part of herself—and we must understand this alienation as the fundamental source of obsessive suffering. With the movement away from the "feminine," feeling side of her nature, Ellen has lost that mystical passion which made her at home in nature and gave her such a rapturous relatedness to "life and joy," filling her with "strength and hope," a "consuming thirst to learn," and offering her finally a wondering glimpse into the "secret of the universe." Now that she has driven her passion away, where shall she feel at home? To what shall she aspire? She has lost her soul; and in exchange for it she has taken up this demonic obsession, a struggle constantly to shame and mortify and break the body, in which this soul is still stirring, but now in purely negative terms. Now, personified by her hunger for food, this old longing for fulfillment and meaningful activity has become her "enemy," causing her that "veritable torment when she sits still," making "every nerve in her body quiver." Now that she is no longer directly conscious of this joy and kinship with the natural world, now that she has taken them as her enemy, they must express themselves symptomatically and pathologically through the intensified cravings of her body.

But this elimination of a part of the self must necessarily leave behind a feeling of despair, the record that a meaningful aspect of being has been pushed out of conscious existence and can no longer legitimately strive for its development. In fact, Ellen's despair at this point in her life is beyond doubt. Even at the beginning of her illness, this despair is so acute that it is transformed into a longing for death. But death "no longer appears to her as terrible; death is not a man with the scythe," but as she herself describes it, "a glorious woman, white asters in her dark hair, large eyes, dream-deep and gray." This image of death is a precise personification of her own feminine nature, which she has lost; her longing for death, as woman, is really a longing for reunification with her own, now alienated, feminine self.

The second expression of her despair is her emptiness. She complained of this emptiness throughout her life and suffered it even as a child. Then, too, it held the same meaning—a movement away from the sensual aspects of self, which was reflected in her renunciation of sweets. But from the time the obsession develops, this emptiness becomes far more acute. She writes a poem in which she describes herself as "unfruitful, a discarded shell, cracked, unusable," a "worthless husk." She cries out also from the pages of her diary: "What is the meaning of this terrible feeling of emptiness—the horrible feeling of dissatisfaction which takes hold after each meal? My heart sinks, I feel it bodily, it is an indescribably miserable feeling." To this refrain she returns again and again, always struggling for an understanding she is unable to achieve. "After dinner," she says, "my mood is always at its worst. I would rather not eat at all, so as not to have the horrible feeling after dinner. All day I am afraid of that feeling. How shall I describe it? It is a dull, empty feeling at the heart."

Indeed, we would expect Ellen West to feel more than ever empty after a meal, when it becomes apparent that even food cannot possibly serve as an adequate substitute for that feminine side of existence she has lost. Later in her life her physician comments upon this. "One has less the impression," he says, "that she suffers under a genuine depressive affect than that she feels herself physically empty and dead, completely hollow, and suffers precisely from the fact that she cannot achieve any affect." Is it possible? Ellen West, this passionate girl, can no longer feel? But of course we know that she cannot feel, of course she seems to herself a discarded shell, empty and dead—this woman has progressively retreated from her own soul, from that wonderful inner being of hers, that illogical "I" she spoke of.

From the outset we know that this gifted, passionate woman will never be able to make a simple peace with her conflict by turning her passion into her enemy and attempting to destroy it. For her, the shift to masculine values simply will not be able to work. Her soul will continue to press for expression and existence by filling her with hungers and longings she will not be able to suppress. That is why the *idée fixe* of being thin, which Ellen now develops, is always accompanied by the "compulsion of always having to think about eating."

And here we come upon what may well be the most essential understanding of obsessive suffering. Obsession is, in fact, a drama, in which that inner being one has hoped to dominate and control keeps struggling to return. The obsession expresses both the *will to destroy* this self, by mortifying the body and starving the flesh, and the *longing to be reunited with it,* through the eating up of food. It is only in terms of this fundamental ambivalence that we can understand the symptoms and the profound contradictions of the obsessive struggle, which claimed the life of Ellen West.

It is, in fact, impossible to cease yearning for a part of the self, impossible to drive it away, to mourn and be done with mourning, and then to forget it. We remain fundamentally whole, and therefore, whatever is driven from conscious experience continues to live a life of its own, transformed now perhaps, unrecognizable, sometimes pictured as a feminine figure of death, sometimes experienced as a terrible longing, a yearning, a hunger, but now with its focus narrowed, its object more literal and concrete. Now Ellen West longs for food where she formerly longed for life and fulfillment and the radiant joy of existence. Thus, Ellen speaks of the "fabulous, *sweet* land of life," as if it were a luscious fruit she could pluck and put into her mouth. Similarly, when she feels a moment of brief reprieve from her obsession she says that she could "feel something *sweet* in my breast," as if her old, lost inner being had now returned and could be tasted in all its power of nourishment. She talks about it being "sweet to fear and to suffer, to grow and to become," as if she is fated ever to associate this "illogical I" in all its yearnings and aspirations, with those sweets she renounced already in childhood.

In the metaphoric equation forged by Ellen West, a preoccupation with the body has taken the place of a fascination with the soul. But now we see that hunger has come to take the place of spiritual longing and that food has become the substitute for all other objects of desire. That is why Ellen West develops such a tormented craving to eat; why, as she says, "the thought of eating never leaves her." For eating has become her only link to the feeling and passion she has been struggling with for her entire life. Thus, when we hear that "each day she consumes several pounds of tomatoes and twenty oranges," we realize that this fruit (which stands symbolically for the roundness and fullness of female existence, with all its sweetness and capacity to ripen and grow), must have promised to give her back that inner being she has so ardently longed to destroy.

The demonic quality of obsessive longing arises from the fact that human beings cannot bear this alienation from an essential part of the self. Indeed, the greater this alienation becomes, the greater also becomes the hunger for what has been lost, until at last all that we have hoped to escape is yoked to us through our growing compulsion, our craving and appetite for it. Thus, Ellen West confesses: "When I open my eyes in the morning, my great misery stands before me. Even before I am entirely awake I think of—eating." Soon indeed every hour between meals is filled with the thought, "When shall I get hungry again? Would I perhaps even like to eat something now? And what?"

If only Ellen had been able to answer this question, to break through finally to the idea that she was hungering for a state of being, a unified condition of the self, rather than for a piece of food. Indeed, this girl, unresting in her efforts to understand, does finally come upon the awareness that food cannot satisfy the real nature of her longing. "I even dread," she writes, "to go into the grocery store. The sight of the groceries awakens longings in me which they [the groceries] can never still. It is as though a person tried to quench his thirst with ink."

Ironically enough, the hunger and thirst from which Ellen West suffered would have been more readily quenched with ink. It is a pity she did not understand what her own imagery was trying to tell her. For she, as a writer, required precisely the exercise of her creative capacity if she was to still the craving which expressed itself through her compulsive appetite for food. In the absence of this understanding, however, her life could only be filled by that sense of dread which is known also to every woman struggling with obsession. "Everything in me trembles with dread," she says, "dread of the adders of my everyday, which would coil about me with their cold bodies and press the will to fight out of me. But my exuberant force offers resistance. I shake them off, I must shake them off. The morning must come after this siege of nightmares."

Nowhere, perhaps, is the acute ambivalence of obsession more evident than here. For the object of dread is constantly changing. In one moment she is afraid of those "adders" of conventionality which are killing off her exuberant force. But in the next moment she is terrified of all manifestations of that life-force itself. She writes: "This is the horrible part of my life. It is filled with dread. Dread of eating, dread of hunger, dread of the dread. Only death can save me from this dread."

The longer she lives with her obsession, without managing to understand the real conflict in which she is engaged, the more terrible this conflict grows. When the body continues to feel, although it is starved and driven on long hikes, when she continues to desire, although she is attempting to eliminate desire in herself, the impression must also grow that she is inhabited by an alien presence. And so she cries out: "I am fighting against uncanny powers which are stronger than I. I cannot seize and grasp them."

From this point we must expect to encounter a continual decline. Once the urge for self-development has been made alien, her fear of this enemy must constantly grow. Because of this fear she must intensify the punitive, controlling measures she takes against this "uncanny power." And now her preoccupation with it must also increase, for nothing seems to be able to extirpate it, to starve it finally out of existence, to purge it from its claim upon her existence. Soon, therefore, Ellen becomes more and more debilitated, goes back to bed in the afternoon, and is terribly tortured by the feeling that "her instincts are stronger than her reason."

But this is the girl who lived in her instincts; never completely at peace there, never without conflict, but with a mighty will for joy and vocation. This is the girl who longed to transform the world. And who now has lost all world but this futile and tragic struggle to destroy her soul.

We know, however, that there is a force of nature, of sensual striving, which cannot be permanently suppressed, or even permanently directed into these misleading symbolic channels. The very giftedness of Ellen West, the sincerity of her struggle to understand, is a sure guarantee that nature will continue to reassert itself and attempt to heal her. Even late in her life, when she is in the sanatorium, she feels a "stirring" inside of herself, her old passion reawakening, a "turmoil and ferment," as if her soul were coming alive again. She speaks now of bringing to light "what lies buried and hidden in me." And now, when she can allow this stirring to enlarge itself and to develop, when "a spiritual relaxation sets in," we find that she will eat anything that is put before her, "including things she has not touched in years: soup, potatoes, meats, sweet dishes, chocolate."

Permission for sensual indulgence is invariably accompanied by an awakening of Ellen's old ambition and desire to learn; for these, which we ordinarily think of as opposites—our sensual pleasures and our intellectual joys—belong in fact to the same feminine principle that is returning to Ellen now. And so, as she begins in the sanatorium to eat soup and potatoes, she also begins to attend lectures at the university. She takes notes "with great concentration," speaks of being reborn, and now, too, her body becomes larger and there comes finally a night when she writes: "As soon as I close my eyes there come poems, poems, poems. If I wanted to write them all down I should have to fill pages and pages—hospital poems . . . weak and full of inner restraint. They only beat their wings softly; but at least something is STIRRING. God grant that it may grow."

It can be no accident that her imagery for this rebirth is borrowed from nature, from the organic, vegetative world. It is a question now of things that grow and ripen and stir. It is an imagery suggestive also of the oldest iconography for the soul, the butterfly, symbol of rebirth, of joy and bliss. Now, when she wakes at night, she finds it "beautiful to be awake." Her heart throbs, and there is something sweet she says in her breast, "which wants to grow and become."

These words were written four months before Ellen West committed suicide. Even then, in the sanatorium, while doctors were diagnosing an incurable condition for which there was no hope, when her illness was so terribly advanced she lived in constant agitation and dread, this life-giving aspiration, this sense of sweetness, this longing to take up her own development came back to her again, and showed her the way beyond her obsessive suffering, by giving her the experience of creative wholeness for which we hunger.

But Ellen West, who has brought us to this essential knowledge of obsession, did not survive. The morning after she wrote of her spiritual rebirth, the stirring of new life had already vanished. She awoke the next day with sadness and with again a feeling of terrible hunger. After all those years, during which she had sided with the masculine aspects of her being, she could not now permit herself this feast of rapture for more than a single night.

The rest we know. The way she left the sanatorium and returned to her family. The way there, too, after an initial period of crisis, the soul again returned. Once again, she ate butter and sugar, chocolate creams, and Easter eggs; she read Goethe and Rilke, took walks, wrote letters. And then, later, as she went alone into her room, and found that once again she was in terrible conflict, afraid of this sensual and spiritual pleasure she had just allowed to herself, she sat down on her bed and took a large amount of fatal poison. If she could not live out her appetite for life, it yet remained within her power to strike a final, mortal blow against that appetite and to strike away from herself forever the dangerous stirring of her own hungry, passionate soul.

So I have imagined her, like some great and tragic heroine, defeated finally by that very division of being that afflicts her entire culture. Indeed, it was only a few months before her death that Ellen West wrote the words: "I feel myself quite passively the stage on which two hostile forces are mangling each other." Now, one of these forces, which in our culture we call the masculine, has won out.

The story of Ellen West is no less than the drama of the defeat and impoverishment of the female soul, from which we, in our own day, who suffer from obsession, also suffer. This finally is the ancient warfare we, too, enact as we pursue our hatred of the body. But we, if we require consolation for this tragic tale, may comfort ourselves with the reflection that the life and the death of Ellen West are redeemed through us when she becomes for us the means to understanding and liberation. And even more—by the fact that in her living and dying she bore such passionate witness that these two, apparently primordial enemies, the body and the soul, are really one.

16. ALMA, THE SOUL

> The human's basic biological need to eat cannot be separated from symbols and metaphors of . . . feasting, social and kin relations, and sacred ritual. —Peter Farb and George Armelagos

> Dinnertime came and the men returned to eat. The table was laid out under the tall cedar trees on long boards supported by sawhorses. Something seemed to stir in the blood of the men and women. Bonds of ownership were dropped or openly flouted. . . . Everyone seemed to hover close to some tantalizing, communal racial memory. —Agnes Smedley, *Daughter of Earth*

THE CURTAIN CLOSES. For a long, long moment we are unable to leave the theater. We sit in our seats, shaken with recognition. It is the drama of our own hidden lives we have seen enacted here. Like Ellen West and all the anorexic girls of our own time, like all the women climbing onto a scale this morning, and all the women taking too many laxatives tonight, we too have proved to be submissive, eager to please the culture of our fathers, through the mastery of our bodies and the sacrifice of all the hungers of our soul.

But do I mean this literally? Do I believe that today, in the last quarter of the twentieth century, we women of a materialist culture are really engaged in a battle about the soul?

I have, indeed, come upon an unexpected confirmation that this is so. For Hilde Bruch, the psychiatrist, also arrives at the very parable we have been discussing. In an effort to conceal the identity of her anorexic patient she names her Alma. And we may happen to recall that the Latin word for Alma means soul. Thus, if we transcribe this passage, placing the word "soul" where the name Alma appears, what we read becomes indeed a symbolic account of the soul's impoverishment.

> At fifteen the soul had been healthy and well-developed, had menstruated at age twelve, was five feet six inches tall and weighed one hundred twenty pounds. At that time the soul's mother urged her to change to a school with higher academic standing, a change she resisted; her father suggested that she should watch her weight, an idea that she took up with great eagerness, and she began a rigid diet. . . . That she could be thin gave her a sense of pride, power, and accomplishment. Whatever low point her weight reached, the soul feared that she might become "too fat" if she gained as little as an ounce. There was also a marked change in her character and behavior. Formerly sweet, obedient, and considerate, the soul became more and more demanding, obstinate, irritable and arrogant.
>
> When she came for consultation, the soul looked like a walking skeleton . . . with her legs sticking out like broomsticks, every rib showing, and her shoulder blades standing up like little wings.
>
> Her mother mentioned, "when I put my arms around her I feel nothing but bones, like a frightened little bird." The soul's arms and legs were covered with soft hair, her complexion had a yellowish tint, and her dry hair hung down in strings. Most striking was the face of the soul—hollow like that of a shriveled-up old woman with a wasting disease, sunken eyes, a sharply pointed nose. . . . When she spoke or smiled . . . one could see every movement of the muscles around her mouth and eyes, like an animated anatomical representation of the skull.[1]

Thus, we come face-to-face with a woman's soul in this last quarter of the twentieth century. Hollow, shriveled-up, suffering from a wasting disease, with shrunken eyes and sharply pointed nose, converted from a principle of joy to a doomed conqueror of nature, the soul has revealed the hidden demonism of this retreat from the female, this struggle against the flesh. It has become a death mask, a grinning skull, pleased with its conquest, stubbornly denying that it is ill. And when Alma, the soul, says: "I enjoy having this disease and I want it. I cannot convince myself that I am sick and that there is anything from which I have to recover," we must confront this confession of complicity. But what a terrible substitute this anorexic soul is for the female soul we might have if we were permitted to claim it. For in that female soul, which is not starving itself to death, there must be hiding all that the dominant culture has driven away from itself. Joy, ecstasy, a feeling of worship, powerful emotion, passion, pleasure in the body, kinship with nature, a knowledge of the animal self and all that unspoken music of existence this soul would sing.

And so finally we understand that when Alma, our soul, is starving herself to death, what she needs to be given to feed her hunger is a reentry into the positive knowledge of woman's experience. How often, therefore, I have found myself wishing that Alma might one day be invited to attend an event like the Dinner Party given by Judy Chicago, where thirty-nine women of symbolic meaning and accomplishment have also been invited to dine, their places set out at three long tables placed together in an equilateral triangle and covered with linen cloths.*

I do not know, of course, whether Judy Chicago intended the full range of meaning I perceive in this symbolic gathering, but I can imagine how this spiritual banquet might be profoundly healing to Alma, who would meet here an important, cultural expression of woman's rediscovered power and joy. I can imagine also how the whole history of this project might affect her, helping her to discover another vision of discipline and will and how they are compatible with food and eating together and laughter. Indeed, it can be no accident that in this time of obsession with woman's hunger and size, a cultural event takes place celebrating all the female qualities that the dominant culture suppresses or denies.

At this feast of souls we might hope that Alma would begin to discover her own true nature again as she gazes at these ceramic

*This project has been exhibited in various museums throughout the country. I saw it in San Francisco. For readers who have not been able to see it, I recommend *The Dinner Party*, by Judy Chicago, Garden City, 1979.

representations of the female vulva, through which the whole range of our spiritual accomplishment as women is expressed—our capacity to think, to act, to struggle, to cry out, to express, to give birth to ourselves anew in the sign of that female principle through which the body is known as the altogether fitting and wholesome habitation of the soul.

I can imagine further, how little by little, as she walks along these tables, from plate to plate, a deeper sense of symbolic meaning might make its way to her—a feeling that she has been called to partake of the very power that is being celebrated here. For it would, I feel sure, become apparent to her that these poets and scholars and noblewomen and former slaves and Indian guides and painters and astronomers have not been invited here merely to dine. They are the feast that is being served up to her, on these ceremonial plates that invite us to eat and to take into ourselves again the lost and alienated powers of our own kind.

And then, as she sits down to this totem meal, where she is encouraged to know and express all those expansive, devouring urges of her own being and to hunger for and to crave her own enlargement as a woman, she will enter into a positive vision of woman and be able finally to forgive this body which bears, in its fullness and swelling, in its odors of musk and sex and unimaginable permissions for sensual pleasure, her own possibility of reconciliation with her sensuality and with the whole female side of existence. And then her retreat from the female will be transformed into celebration. And poor, emaciated Alma, who is happy to be ill, can take her place eating and drinking in this great tableau of affirmation, dappled with shadow and light, and there is all that rejoicing, presided over by an immense, untrammeled, and expansive laughter.

NOTES

1. CONFESSIONS OF AN EATER

1. June Jordan, *Passion,* Boston, 1980.
2. Jean Cocteau, *Opium: The Diary of a Cure,* London, 1957.
3. Ibid.
4. James Hillman, *The Dream and the Underworld,* New York, 1979.

2. THE FLESH AND THE DEVIL

1. Sally Hegelson, *TWA Ambassador,* July 1980.
2. Private communication.
3. Private communication.
4. Susan Griffin, *Woman and Nature: The Roaring Inside Her,* New York, 1978.

3. THE SKEPTIC

1. *San Francisco Examiner Chronicle,* December 27, 1980.
2. Ibid.
3. *Harvard Medical School Health Letter,* Vol. 41, No. 2, December 1980.
4. Margaret MacKenzie, "The Politics of Body Size: Fear of Fat," Pacifica Tape Library, Los Angeles, 1980.
5. Dr. George Mann, "The Influence of Obesity on Health," *New England Journal of Medicine,* July–August 1974.
6. Phyllis Lehmann, "Your Choice: Breast Reshaping," *Vogue,* July 1979.
7. Kitty Kelly, *The Glamour Spas,* New York, 1976.
8. *San Francisco Chronicle,* January 17, 1981
9. *Harvard Medical School Health Letter,* loc. cit.
10. Susie Orbach, *Fat Is a Feminist Issue: The Anti-Diet Guide to Permanent Weight Loss,* New York, 1978.
11. MacKenzie, "The Politics of Body Size."
12. Gloria Heidi, *Winning the Age Game,* Garden City, N.Y. 1976.
13. Ibid.

13. Ibid.
14. Orbach, *Fat Is a Feminist Issue.*
15. Stanley H. Title, Weight Control Dynamics, New York.
16. A. W. Ferriss, Medical Weight Reduction, San Francisco, Calif.
17. Professional Weight Control, Ltd., Overland Park, Kansas
18. Ruthe Stein, "How Betty Sausa Lost 79 Pounds," and "Surgery for the Obese," *San Francisco Chronicle,* September 1, 1979.
19. Hilde Bruch, *Eating Disorders,* New York, 1973.
20. MacKenzie, "The Politics of Body Size".
21. Hilde Bruch, *The Golden Cage,* New York, 1979.
22. Heidi, *Winning the Age Game.*
23. *West Point Fitness and Diet Book.*
24. Robert Linn, *The Last Chance Diet Book,* New York, 1976.
25. Ibid.
26. St. John, "Exhortation to Theodore," in Katherine M. Rogers, *The Troublesome Helpmate: A History of Misogyny in Literature,* Seattle, Washington, 1966.
27. Linn, *The Last Chance Diet Book.*
28. J. Huizinga, *The Waning of the Middle Ages,* Garden City, N.Y., 1954.

4. THE HUNGER ARTIST

1. Hilde Bruch, *The Golden Cage: The Enigma of Anorexia Nervosa,* New York, 1978.
2. Aimee Liu, *Solitaire,* New York, 1979.
3. Sandra Gilbert, "Hunger Pains," *University Publishing,* Fall 1979.
4. Bruch, *Golden Cage.*
5. Ibid.
6. Franz Kafka, "The Hunger Artist," *Selected Stories of Franz Kafka,* New York, 1952.
7. Private communication.
8. Marcia Millman, *Such a Pretty Face,* New York, 1980.
9. Private correspondence.

5. THE OLDEST CULTURAL ISSUE

1. Norman O. Brown, *Life Against Death: The Psychoanalytical Meaning of History,* New York, 1959.
2. Julian Jaynes, *The Origins of Consciousness in the Breakdown of the Bicameral Mind,* Boston, 1976.
3. Rogers, *The Troublesome Helpmate.*
4. Edward Conze, *Buddhism: Its Essence and Development,* New York, 1959.

5. Ibid.
6. Ernest Becker, *The Denial of Death,* New York, 1975.
7. Ibid.
8. Millman, *Such a Pretty Face.*
9. MacKenzie, "The Politics of Body Size."
10. Maria Brenner, "Bulmarexia," *Savvy,* June 6, 1980.
11. Gilbert, "Hunger Pains."
12. Bruch, *The Golden Cage.*

6. SISTERS

1. *Edible Woman,* Boston, 1969.
2. Ibid.
3. Ibid.
4. Margaret Atwood, *Lady Oracle,* New York, 1976.
5. Ibid.
6. Margaret Laurence, *The Fire Dwellers,* New York, 1969.

7. THE MATRIARCH

1. Nor Hall, *The Moon and the Virgin,* New York, 1980.
2. Ibid.
3. J. J. Bachofen in Hall, ibid.
4. Hall, ibid.
5. Ibid.
6. Atwood, *Lady Oracle.*
7. Hall, *The Moon and the Virgin.*
8. Anne Tucker, *Woman's Eye,* New York, 1973.
9. Dorothea Lange, *Photos,* New York, 1966.
10. Karen Petersen and J. J. Wilson, *Women Artists: Recognition and Reappraisal from the Early Middle Ages to the Twentieth Century,* New York, 1976.
11. Ibid.
12. Gillian Perry, *Paula Modersohn-Becker,* New York, 1978.
13. Ibid.
14. Kenneth Clark, *Nude: A Study of Ideal Form,* New York, 1956.

8. THE BOUTIQUE

1. Hilde Bruch, *Eating Disorders: Obesity, Anorexia Nervosa, and the Person Within,* New York, 1973.
2. Brenner, "Bulmarexia."
3. Susan Strasberg, *Bitter Sweet,* New York, 1980.

4. *GEO,* April 1980.

5. Morey Stanyan on Carole Shaw, *San Francisco Examiner Chronicle,* January 20, 1980.

6. Bruch, *Eating Disorders.*

7. Griffin, *Woman and Nature.*

8. *This Week in Review, San Francisco Examiner Chronicle,* October 5, 1980; "December," December 4, 1980.

9. Norman Mailer, *Marilyn: A Biography,* New York, 1973.

10. Strasberg, *Bitter Sweet.*

9. WHY NOW?

1. Louise Bernikow, *Among Women,* New York, 1980.

2. Jana Harris, *Manhattan as a Second Language,* Harper & Row, forthcoming.

3. Bruch, *The Golden Cage.*

4. Liu, *Solitaire.*

5. Ibid.

6. Bruch, *The Golden Cage.*

7. Ibid.

8. Liu, *Solitaire.*

9. Heidi, *Winning the Age Game.*

10. Florence Rush, "Pornography: Who Is Hurt?" in *Take Back the Night,* ed. L. Lederer.

11. Ibid.

12. Ibid.

13. Louise Armstrong, *Kiss Daddy Goodnight: A Speak-Out on Incest,* New York, 1978.

14. Grace Paley, review of *The Best Kept Secret* by Florence Rush, *Ms.,* January 1981.

15. Ibid.

10. MAN AND WIFE

1. "Sunday Punch," *San Francisco Examiner Chronicle,* March 2, 1980.

2. Roslyn Lacks, *Woman and Judaism,* Garden City, N.Y., 1980.

3. Bruno Bettelheim, *Symbolic Wounds: Puberty Rites and the Envious Male,* New York, 1962.

4. Beth Trier, *San Francisco Examiner Chronicle,* 1980.

5. *Revelations: Diaries of Women,* ed. Mary J. Moffat and Charlotte Painter, New York, 1975.

6. Lacks, *Woman and Judaism.*
7. Bruch, *Eating Disorders.*
8. Millman, *Such a Pretty Face.*

11. CLUES

1. Friedrich W. Nietzsche, *The Genealogy of Morals,* Garden City, N.Y., 1956.
2. Johann W. von Goethe, *Faust,* trans. Bayard Taylor, New York, 1962.
3. William Faulkner, *Light in August,* New York, 1972.
4. Susan Griffin, *Pornography and Silence: Culture's Revenge Against Nature,* New York, 1981.
5. Wolfgang Lederer, *Fear of Women,* New York, 1968.
6. Ibid.
7. Ibid.

12. THE PRIMORDIAL FEMALE

1. M. Mahler, *On Human Symbiosis and the Vicissitudes of Individuation,* New York, 1968; Dorothy Dinnerstein, *The Mermaid and the Minotaur: Sexual Arrangements and Human Malaise,* New York, 1967; N. Chaderow, *The Reproduction of Mothering,* Berkeley, 1978; Michael Balint, *Primary Love and Psychoanalytic Technique,* London, 1935.
2. *Georgia O'Keeffe: A Portrait by Alfred Stieglitz,* New York, 1976.
3. Erich Neumann, *The Great Mother: An Analysis of the Archetype,* trans. Ralph Manheim, New York, 1963.
4. Dinnerstein, *The Mermaid and the Minotaur.*
5. Becker, *The Denial of Death.*

13. BOY AND GIRL

1. Bruch, *The Golden Cage.*
2. *Anne Frank: The Diary of a Young Girl,* New York, 1967.
3. Ibid.

14. THE MYSTERIOUS CASE OF ELLEN WEST

1. All the quotations in this chapter, unless otherwise noted, are from the diary of Ellen West and are cited by Ludwig Binswanger in "The Case of Ellen West," in *Existence: A New Dimension in Psychiatry and Psychology,* ed. Rollo May, New York, 1958.
2. Virginia Woolf, *A Room of One's Own,* New York, 1957.

15. THE OBSESSION

1. Anzia Yezierska, *The Open Cage,* New York, 1979.
2. Anzia Yezierska, *The Bread Givers,* New York, 1975.

16. ALMA, THE SOUL

1. Bruch, *The Golden Cage.*